I0165152

BREAKING FREE FROM CHRONIC PAIN

HOW I OVERCAME CHRONIC PAIN AND RECLAIMED MY LIFE

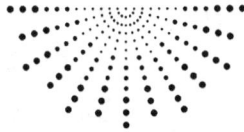

LILI ROAD

LIBRARY TALES PUBLISHING

To my children, to Camille, and to my loved ones.
To all those I've crossed paths with on the road,
I have received from you much more than I could ever
offer in return. You have given meaning to my life.

To all those who have entrusted me with their
sufferings, I hope this book will restore your faith
in life. It can remain beautiful despite everything.
Never lose hope; your best life is yet to come.

INTRODUCTION

Triumphantly emerging from a fierce two-year battle against chronic lower back pain, my sole desire today is to share the keys to my recovery with those who continue to suffer. Now that I am healed, spreading awareness about the mind–body connection (MBC) method that saved me has become a clear and undeniable responsibility I must embrace. If I can make even a small contribution to the structure of healing chronic pain, then it is my duty to do so.

This testimony also aligns with the promise I made to myself after surviving ten years of severe anorexia: One day, I will do something to help those who cannot free themselves from the grip of their demons. At the time, my bold idea was to create support centers abroad. I envisioned places where individuals suffering from eating disorders (ED) could experience a transformative "Canadian break"—a change of environment, a complete escape from daily life, and the healing fulfillment that comes through art. It was this combination that allowed me to overcome my struggles.

Chronic pain is an invisible disease that gnaws at the soul, gradually, insidiously, and inexorably destroying its host. As the horizons of my life narrowed more each day, I became nothing more than a shadow of myself—a hollow shell. Or rather, a shell so full it eventually broke. These physical and psychological pains took many forms: EDs, migraines, recurrent chronic tendinitis in various parts of my body, inexplicable pain, loss of voice, lower back pain, neck pain ... These conditions reappeared periodically, and, as traditional medicine found no apparent physical cause, they were deemed incurable.

"You have to learn to live with it, Miss!"

These words marked my life, often dictating it. Yet, after almost six months of relentless research, I discovered that the key to these afflictions had been within me all along. Unknowingly, I was my own therapy.

This book is my humble testimony, written to tell you: never, ever give up. It's not easy, but chronic pain does not have to be inevitable. We know its causes, and we can heal from it.

When you've just performed a concert and your audience tells you that you brought them joy and happiness—that, for a moment, they forgot about their illness—what magic, what pride, what an honor! Even though it sometimes meant waking up at three in the morning to hit the road, I never doubted why I was doing it. My audiences gave me a true sense of purpose.

Life has meaning when it has meaning.

That's why giving up writing and abruptly leaving the troubadour life contributed to my vertiginous fall. When I expressed my emotions healthily—through outlets like sports or art—I kept my chronic pain at bay. For fifteen years on the road as a performing artist and art therapist, I observed, absorbed, and composed music, inspired by the admirable resilience of the extraordinary people I met along the way. Throughout this book, you'll find the lyrics of my songs woven into its pages. Sharing my most intimate emotions with my audience was like offering myself unmasked, vulnerable, and unarmed.

I still have disc degeneration to this day, but the haunting serenade of pain has ceased. I am finally living again. Pain no longer reigns as a dictator over my existence. I hope my story inspires you to believe that anything is possible. From an anorexic, dropout teenager to a thriving artist and entrepreneur, I seized every opportunity life offered me.

Even though I've changed names to preserve the anonymity of some individuals, I will narrate the seasons of my life with honesty and authenticity. If life inflicted this two-year ordeal on me, perhaps it was so that I could write this book and tell my story. If you are one of the 51 million Americans suffering from chronic pain, I hope my testimony convinces you that permanently freeing yourself from its grip is possible.

CHAPTER ONE

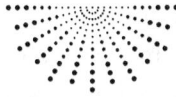

As far back as I can remember, I had a happy childhood—I was the daughter of loving parents and lacked nothing. My father worked hard in our family business, navigating demanding suppliers and increasingly difficult-to-satisfy customers. My mother, a preschool teacher with three little ones, juggled Easter bunnies made of crepe paper and pre-reading preparations. I experienced plentiful vacations, leisure, sports, and other activities with a carefree spirit.

The life of an only child, however, is not always fun. With no siblings—and with my mom's frequent migraines—I rarely had someone to play (or argue) with. So, I invented: I played Monopoly alone with my imaginary friends and played teacher with my teddy bears. One day, barely knee-high, I climbed onto the living room table with a microphone in hand to passionately sing "A Bailar Calypso" by Elli Medeiros in front of an imaginary audience. It felt incredible.

Growing up on folk, rock, and country standards, I started humming Joan Baez, the Beatles, and Elton John at an early age. My emerging passion for music soon became evident.

By middle school, I was considered different and, therefore, strange—quickly becoming a victim of bullying, which eventually forced my parents to homeschool me for over five years. To occupy my days, after finishing my homework, I sang, danced, and wrote—not yet songs, but poems, detective stories, and pages upon pages in my diary. This hobby and passion became my lifeline, especially as I faced the anorexia that gradually crept into my teenage years.

As the years went by, I still didn't know where music would lead me, but it remained my most faithful companion. From charity choirs to musicals on French and Canadian stages, and performances in English pubs and German biergartens, music became more than an escape—it became my reason for being.

I always strived to give my best and share my experiences as a harassed and anorexic teenager. I wanted to evoke emotions in others. It wasn't long before I had a songwriting revelation: During my stay in Canada as a participant in the Rotary Club exchange program, I borrowed a guitar from one of my host fathers and began scribbling notes, chords, and lyrics. This is how "Seize the Day," my very first song, was born. Through this process, I began to understand that everything I had experienced thus far had meaning. The personal trials I had overcome, with the help of music, brought me to where I am today and shaped who I've become. The road I've taken has been winding and filled with obstacles, but these challenges have shown me the true power of music and art: the power to build and rebuild oneself.

When I returned from Canada, I continued my studies in applied foreign languages and later enrolled in business school. I wanted to ensure that even if I gave up on singing as a profession, my degrees would allow me to find a position where I could speak English and travel the world. During this time, I also continued singing in several bands—and sometimes alone with my guitar. I was not yet "Lili Road" the artist, but my audience—the stage of life and anyone and everyone around me—was already present. Finally, I began to feel at home.

CHAPTER TWO

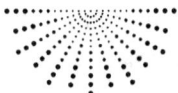

*I*n June 2005, armed with my diplomas, my professional life began with a fulfilling career as a buyer, leading me to many corners of the world. But during this time, I also began regularly posting videos of my original songs on YouTube. Before I knew it, my passion for music began to take precedence over everything else, urging me to change the direction of my life. Thus, Lili Road the artist was officially born—named after "Lili," the nickname given to me by my grandmother as a child, and "Road," symbolizing my love of traveling far and wide to share my passion with others.

We may not be family, but my heart always trusted you
I didn't know you'd lead me so far, so far on that winding
* road …*
I didn't know you would change my life … in a way, in
* a way.*

Ten years have already gone by … so fast …
And what a decade it's been
And what a cavalcade it's been,

But it feels like only yesterday.

Now we've been apart for so long, but nothing has changed
  in my heart,
You became just family, where a part of me belongs
I didn't know I would feel this way ... in a way, in a way.
Now, I am back here lost for words, just hope you can be
  proud of me,
Let my gratitude be heard for all that you guys did for me,
I didn't know I would love you so ... in a way, in a way.

With the loss of Sandra, my host mother, in April 2021, an entire chapter of my life crumbled. I felt an overwhelming gratitude for the privilege of knowing her, but I also felt the weight of precious memories vanishing with her. Sandra—who always believed in me. Sandra—who urged me to cling to my dreams. Sandra—who advised me to follow the signs destiny placed on my path. Because of Sandra, that's exactly what I did: after her passing, I threw myself even deeper into the world of music. I appeared on radio and TV shows, collaborated with many talented musicians, and performed three hundred concerts a year. Largely thanks to Sandra, my passion was finally being expressed live.

Through some charitable events I participated in, I discovered that music could build bridges and profoundly impact children with autism and other developmental disabilities. This revelation led me to a new challenge: embarking on the journey of obtaining a degree in art therapy at the Free Faculty of Medicine of Lille. I had the immense privilege of gaining experience in the pediatric surgery and orthopedics operating rooms at the University Hospital of Lille. At the time, introducing art therapy into an operating room was met with resistance. However, thanks to Dr. É. Nectoux and M. O. Hanssens, who advocated on my behalf, I was able to demonstrate through my thesis the effectiveness of art therapy in managing pain in children before and after surgery.

Freshly graduated, I founded **Music & Motion**. Yet, the most beautiful victory of all came one Saturday morning in the form of a phone call. A moved mother informed me that her son Hugo—one of the little boys I was treating, who has autism and was non-speaking— had spoken his first words: "Lili" and "guitar." The news brought tears to my eyes. I was overwhelmed with intense emotion and deeply grateful for the opportunity to care for this young boy.

In a few words, my life was both active and fulfilling—my family and professional lives moving at full speed.

Until one day in late 2021, when the storm suddenly broke.

PART I
MY AUTUMN DRAGS ON

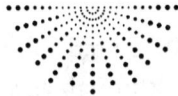

Wounds and burns, etchings on my skin,
Tales whispered by each scar's radiant sheen.

Hard blows, your flaws, vices profound,
Where obscure sorrows gleam, where dark sorrows
    sound.

So live your life and don't just dream your dreams,
And live your dreams—don't merely drift life's streams.

Vacancies and cruelties, inked tattoos, we all know,
No chances, pure intents, through ages we sow.

Lessons to gather, lessons to bestow,
The pain we carry shapes the seeds we grow.

So live your life and don't just dream your dreams,
And live your dreams—don't merely drift life's streams.

No divine entwining here—all you earn, owed only
    to you,
And as they say, such is life, through and through.

So live your life and don't just dream your dreams,
And live your dreams—don't merely drift life's streams.

CHAPTER THREE

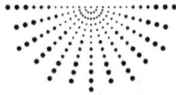

*I*t's September 2021, 6:00 a.m. on a Friday. The fatigue from the week is starting to take its toll—both at work and at home—and I still need to summon the energy to teach my students and take care of the kids. I am an English professor and the Dean of an international professional program, with numerous deadlines looming. Adding to this is the early onset of parental burnout: nights with my one-year-old, Emily, are anything but peaceful. Her father, Camille, lives an hour away with his other children, of whom he has alternating custody, and he only joins us on weekends.

Cam and I knew the weeks would be challenging, but we were determined to fully live our dream of building a big, beautiful, blended family. The energy and drive that brought us together led us to believe we could handle it all seamlessly. After all, it was only supposed to be temporary.

But our weekend reunions rarely live up to the romantic fantasy we hope for. The days demand the flawless coordination of three to five children. Between groceries, transportation, homework, and Cam's travels across France to coach a hockey team, weekends are overwhelming. We're a "variable geometry family," as I like to call us, and it's challenging for everyone to find their place in a household with common rules but vastly different lifestyles.

> **Born from a dream, a wild desire's flare,**
> **Yet daily life gnaws at them, unaware.**
> **Born of hearts yearning, in this dance they weave,**
> **Where they, in compromise, choose love to believe.**
> **Yet they love through sunshine and rain.**

Little Emily wakes up almost every hour crying, so sleep has become fragmented and far from restorative. I frequently end up sleeping with her—somehow always balancing on the edge of the bed. During the day, Cam and I are both exhausted. We console ourselves with the thought that her night terrors will eventually fade, the household will stabilize, and she'll find her place. But the weeks pass, and I grow more tired, less capable of coping.

On this September morning, as usual, I wake up slightly before my little one. As I rise, a sharp pain shoots through my lower back. I pause, frightened, but convince myself it's nothing serious. After all, as a long-time runner, I've dealt with morning aches before.

I shake it off and dive into my daily marathon: helping Emily get dressed, preparing her breakfast, persuading her to eat (no small feat), managing the two eldest children, and carving out a sliver of time for myself—if I'm lucky.

Days turn into weeks, and the pain in my back intensifies, slowly engulfing my body. Movements become an ordeal, as dagger-like pains shoot through my lumbar region. I try every over-the-counter remedy —heating patches, cooling creams, pills, tablets—yet nothing works.

Despite advice from family and colleagues, I stubbornly refuse to consult my doctor. *It's just a simple backache; it'll go away,* I tell myself. I refuse to admit I can no longer bend forward, sit, or stand for more than ten minutes. I act as though nothing is wrong, believing that denial will somehow make the pain more bearable.

Months later, at my breaking point, I finally see my doctor. He prescribes anti-inflammatories and recommends heating cream. He's unconcerned and assures me it will improve with rest. But rest? When? How?

Born from little habits they've always known,
Yet no strength left to endure; they've outgrown.
Born from life's relentless, demanding quest,
In its face, they find themselves bereft.

Papers pile up on my desk, administrative tasks accumulate, and I've never been this behind. The university is restructuring, and, like many workplaces, we're constantly expected to do more with less. A new education reform adds to the pressure, with last-minute updates forcing teachers to adapt "very reactively, please," for the students' sake.

And Emily? Do I put her on hold? There's also the groceries, the cleaning, the laundry ... I'm caught in the endless spiral of *"Everything is important, and everything must be done."*

This reasoning held—until the day I was no longer physically or psychologically capable of managing this elusive *everything*. I am just a human being with limits, and, little by little, I've reached them.

I make compromises: I stop all physical activity due to a lack of time, energy, and motivation—a heartbreaking decision. Sports have always been part of my life: tennis, my first love; badminton, discovered during university; and field hockey with my children. Having already given up my artistic career, letting go of sports feels like another piece of myself slipping away.

The days are polluted by constant pain, and my mind is consumed by the desperate need to end it. I am in distress, in survival mode. One weekend, amidst his travels, Cam offers to take over so I can catch a breath at the Citadel of Lille. Unable to run, I drag myself there, hoping for a reprieve. Instead, I return home burdened with new spirals of negative thoughts about my state.

I try going to bed at 8:00 p.m., sacrificing precious moments with my teenagers, Mathilde and Alex, but I have no choice. The year-end celebrations that I once looked forward to approach, bringing more stress than joy. Hiding gifts, decorating the house, baking with my eldest—tasks that should be festive become exhausting.

Life with our blended family had already been tested by the pandemic. Confined at Cam's countryside house during lockdown, we initially managed with precision and optimism. But as weeks passed, anxiety, tension, and the weight of communal living took their toll. A year later, the aftershocks still reverberate.

"Codeine? Opium? Injections? To relieve you, there's nothing left but that, Miss!"

I cry from the stress and anxiety. Emily's insomnia leaves me in a state of constant exhaustion. Vitamins and magnesium no longer suffice. I find myself dozing at my desk or bursting into tears under the weight of it all.

I can't take it anymore. My colleagues try to support me, but they, too, are overwhelmed. The pain never leaves, and I've become a victim of parental and professional burnout. I am, quite literally, at the end of my rope.

CHAPTER FOUR

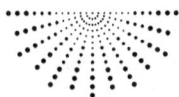

In January 2022, as the new academic term begins, it becomes increasingly clear that I am struggling to balance my responsibilities. Colleagues suggest that I consider taking a break to recover, but I quickly dismiss the idea. *Taking a break? That's not really in my nature.* There's too much to do. At the university, we're short-staffed, and at home, the children need me. A simple backache won't stop me. I must hold on.

Three months of this suffering pass—the official threshold, according to the International Classification of Diseases, for a "chronic pain sufferer." I can no longer put on my socks or lift my daughter into her car seat. My life has been reduced to a constant state of acute pain—a relentless sensation of a bar wedged in my lower back, accompanied by unbearable stabbing pains radiating down my left leg. My optimism wanes a little more each day as I resign myself to living in slow motion. The children live with a weakened mother, and Camille shows signs of fatigue as he tries to overcompensate for my limitations. Although we support each other, our patience with one another begins to erode.

Listening to their tale, like a grimoire's unfold,

Dreams and magic growing cold.

One cold January morning, a stabbing pain in my lower back brings me to my knees. The pain is excruciating, and I resign myself to staying home from work. My general practitioner, seeing my state, puts me on sick leave—something I should have done much earlier. He insists I take care of myself and finally rest. He administers several injections directly into my back and warns me: if I don't act now, the pain will return with a vengeance.

But it does return, and soon I am completely debilitated. Camille juggles an impossible schedule, constantly traveling back and forth, searching for the best (or least bad) solutions. I continue my physiotherapy sessions, but each exercise is agony, even on a high dose of painkillers. Anxiety attacks creep in, and I find myself lashing out at others. Ultimately, I direct most of my resentment inward. I berate myself for being defeated by what I perceive as a "minor" back pain. Regret consumes me: regret for lifting those boxes when I shouldn't have, regret for taking on extra work, regret for never making time for myself.

As I struggle, I become mentally weaker and more susceptible to the weight of others' words—whether well-intentioned or not. My doctors offer little solace. They are evasive about the causes of my pain and especially about the possibility of a cure. Instead of reassuring me, each appointment pulls me further from hope. Over several months, I cycle through various specialists, desperately seeking answers. But traditional medicine offers me little beyond prescriptions for stronger and stronger painkillers. I begin to doubt the existence of a solution and whether the next doctor will be any different from the last.

Unintentionally, everyone around me seems to have an opinion about my pain. Some say, *"You're too focused on yourself! Stop feeling sorry for yourself."* Others offer dismissive comparisons like, *"There are worse things than what you're going through!"* or *"We all have back pain."* Then there are those who smugly remind me, *"You were always told you were doing too much—it was bound to happen."*

And, of course, there's the never-ending stream of unsolicited advice: *"Apply ice! No, use heat!" "Sleep on your back, not your stomach!"*

"Stretch, but not too much!" "Go see my physio, my osteopath, my chiropractor, my podiatrist, my magnetizer, my psychic!" Everyone seems to have a miracle professional who helped their neighbor's sister-in-law's daughter.

We will lay bare all our certainties,
With honesty and heartful keys.
We'll share our truths, open and free,
The real stories, as much as can be.

Weeks pass, and my anger gives way to a deep sense of abandonment. My life feels reduced to an endless series of painful chores. I become passive, lacking the strength to fight back. Desperate for connection, I join a Facebook group where members share anecdotes about their daily struggles with chronic lower back or neck pain.

Many of the group members are in far worse situations: repeated surgeries, worsening pain that has persisted for years, and financial struggles tied to their disability. Their stories terrify me. I am haunted by the thought that this could be my future, too.

CHAPTER FIVE

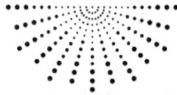

he months pass tirelessly as I drag on alongside my pain—
my new, unwelcome companion. I've been on sick leave for
several months now, and it's weighing heavily on me. In late March, I
receive the results of the MRI my general practitioner prescribed weeks
ago. The verdict is finally in: the imaging reveals, among other things,
the presence of an L5-S1 hernia and disc degeneration at the same
level. To my surprise, I feel ecstatic at the diagnosis. *Finally, the doctors
know what's wrong with me; now they can treat me,* I think.

But my excitement is short-lived. The doctors inform me there's
not much to be done. *Degeneration can't be treated.* I'm told to learn to
live with the pain and advised to give up running or carrying anything
—including my daughter.

Still, a glimmer of resistance sparks in a corner of my mind:
Perhaps I haven't explored all my options yet. I begin hydrotherapy
alongside physiotherapy, but despite the care and medication, I see no
real improvement. Gradually, I am stripped of everything that defines
me: the active, sporty mom who travels and embraces life fully. I
become, in my eyes, nothing more than a chronic pain sufferer. Overcoming pain becomes my sole daily mission, overshadowing everything else. Each failed attempt to live normally feels like a bitter

failure, and the possibility of reclaiming my old life fades a little more each day.

In 1970, Abraham Maslow created a hierarchy of fundamental needs in the form of a pyramid. This psychological theory ranks human needs into five levels: physiological needs, safety, belonging, self-esteem, and self-actualization. The pyramid illustrates how individuals seek to satisfy these needs progressively, from the base to the top, to reach their full potential.

Unfortunately, my chronic pain traps me at the base of this pyramid—at the lowest level of basic physiological needs. This foundation, vital for satisfying higher-level needs, remains unattainable for me. Consequently, the need for safety, characteristic of the next level, also goes unmet. I live in constant insecurity and fear.

My pain also hampers my essential need for autonomy. I want to continue participating in household life, so I push myself to accomplish even the tiniest daily tasks—but it's nearly impossible. Camille rushes around, juggling everything, while becoming a witness to my physical crises, bad moods, and deep despair. I feel ashamed, diminished, and humiliated. I am overwhelmed by the unbearable sensation of being a burden to those around me.

I can't manage the grocery shopping or cleaning. Even getting out of bed or getting dressed is laborious. My heart breaks when I hear my two-year-old daughter say, "Wait, Mummy—I'll help you put on your socks."

How can I envision any long-term projects when getting out of bed feels insurmountable? How can I consider a journey, further education, or any form of self-fulfillment? The very idea seems to have vanished entirely. Gradually, I sink into a deep depression. I am sad, tired, and irritable all the time, consumed day and night by pain and endless spirals of rumination. I lose interest in everything—even reading or watching a good series no longer appeals to me.

Lying down is no relief; the pain is too excruciating. Nothing brings me pleasure anymore. I simply endure my life.

Eventually, I lay down my weapons and resign to my fate completely: Pain has won the game, and I must accept that it will accompany me for the rest of my days.

Like a stream, softly ebbing its flow,
She thinks of it, day in, day out...

A monstrous sense of guilt grows inside me: *Why didn't I act sooner? Why didn't I spare myself this stress?* Darker thoughts creep in: *Is life worth living like this? Would death be gentler?* Sometimes I break down in tears. Other times, the incessant flood of thoughts overwhelms me, and I become completely numb.

Instead of facing what is happening to me in a healthy way, I withdraw into myself. I lose my ability to analyze life's challenges with clarity. Worst-case scenarios dominate my thoughts. When the phone rings, I brace for bad news. Even listening to Camille's anecdotes about his day with his high school students plunges me into helplessness and anxiety.

What used to bring joy now fuels resentment. I envy his ability to experience life while mine is reduced to mere survival. This resentment chips away at our bond, slowly destroying the complicity that once united us. I feel deeply, unbearably alone.

In the weeks that follow, my physical and emotional symptoms worsen. Food becomes a refuge, and I gain weight. I no longer recognize myself. My patience wears thin, and I am prone to fits of anger. My body traps every ounce of tension it can.

Let's hear the warrior's anthem, as the ultimate war
nears,
A solitary life shaped only by the battling of his
fears.

Pain and depression act as magnets, pulling in every aspect of my existence—my attitudes, thoughts, behaviors. They have unpacked their bags and claimed their place as masters of my life. Each day, I wake up asking: *What will they allow me to do today?*

I am nothing more than their devoted servant.

CHAPTER SIX

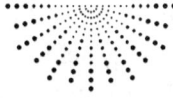

*n April 2022, I seek healing at any cost because I am in pain twenty-four hours a day. I am willing to try anything. I consult doctors in physical medicine and rehabilitation, podiatrists, rheumatologists, physiotherapists, osteopaths, chiropractors … even a renowned magnetizer. Despite returning for several sessions, I notice no improvement. Sometimes, I feel like I'm being taken advantage of by unscrupulous practitioners who keep scheduling appointments, knowing they can't truly help me. Still—*still*—nothing works.

My doctors decide to increase my medication yet again, adding stronger pills to help me sleep. I become a shadow of myself. Patients I meet advise me to "accept things as they are" and rebuild my life around the pain. They suggest I look to them as examples—they've learned to live despite their suffering. But their words, however well-intentioned, only deepen my emotional distress. Far from comforting me, they feel like nails in the coffin of my hope.

As if I don't have enough on my plate, I receive notice of an impending tax audit. Great. Now I need to gather a thousand certificates and papers—yet I can't even sit in a chair without excruciating pain.

Another blow strikes: my two eldest children decide to live with their father. They're tired of living "out of bags" between two homes. I can't blame them. The atmosphere at home has become heavy and anxiety-inducing. They are right to want to protect themselves.

Obsessed with finding a miracle cure, I live in constant fear that my life is ruined—and I cannot let it be. Yet many signs suggest that it already is. The *pain catastrophizing scale*, used by the scientific community to assess perceived pain, its duration, and its impact, reveals the grim reality: empirically, I have hit rock bottom.

Finally, after months of grueling waiting, the long-awaited moment arrives. In June 2022, I join the Back School at the Center of Hope in Villeneuve d'Ascq as a day hospital patient for six weeks. Hope is rekindled within me. I convince myself that these experts hold the long-sought answers to my pain.

I join a group of three other patients. The staff, though dedicated, is visibly overwhelmed and acknowledges they cannot give every patient the attention they deserve. My days fill with hydrotherapy, physiotherapy, therapeutic education, occupational therapy, sophrology, qi gong, and adapted sports activities. Time flies. Rediscovering Nordic walking, light weightlifting, and even holding a badminton racket again revives me. Everything is designed to help me regain confidence in my abilities.

The group dynamic becomes a lifeline. United by a common pain, we develop mutual trust, deep understanding, cooperative solidarity, and genuine empathy. We share our lives as one does with travel companions, knowing we may never see each other again. This collective resilience and beautiful cohesion strengthen us, empowering us to face our challenges.

Yet life's unpredictability strikes twice within our small group. One member loses her brother to a rapid cancer, leaving behind a grieving wife and children. Another member, Thierry, departs the group after only three weeks. Despite his optimism and motivation to reclaim his life after a second arthrodesis, he suffers silently, and the pain ultimately overwhelms him. His absence fills us with sadness, and due to medical confidentiality, we are unable to get any news about him despite our repeated requests.

Being surrounded, cared for, and supported in every aspect of life does wonders for me. I finally focus solely on my recovery. In addition to my usual psychological follow-ups, I attend weekly sessions with the center's psychologist to assess my morale and perception of pain. Looking back, it seems obvious to me that every chronic pain patient should have access to such psychological support. Unfortunately, as with so many places, human resources are insufficient to meet the overwhelming need.

Within days, I notice encouraging signs of improvement. I increase the weights on the machines, my recovery times shorten, and I regain more range of motion in all exercises. The staff acknowledges my progress, both physical and psychological. Functional tests show constant improvement. While the pain persists, new, joyful perspectives begin to emerge. Breaking free from isolation and focusing on myself, I finally glimpse an escape from this living hell. When my mind is calm, my body feels the benefits.

A glimmer of optimism grows within me, reviving my will to fight. By the end of my stay, I consider a gradual return to work starting in September.

The summer holidays approach, and we decide it's too soon to reunite the whole family. So, in July 2022, I spend a week in the mountains with my two teenagers, leaving Emily to enjoy special moments with her father. I cherish moments of well-being with my daughter at a spa overlooking the peaks, surrounded by forty-degree waters. I drive, hike trails, practice yoga, and swim often. In a word, I am reborn.

During this trip, I notice my pain no longer torments me. I feel as though I can finally resume my life where I left it. I make friends with other vacationers while my teenagers frolic with their peers. When they return, we share moments together—moments where they rediscover the mother they once knew: smiling, happy, and content.

Meanwhile, Emily spends a wonderful week camping with her father, swimming in the Atlantic with her dad and brother. Soon, she'll return and tell me all about her adventures. I can't wait to hear her little voice say, "Your back doesn't hurt anymore, Mummy. Will you come with me in the water?"

Our reunion promises to be magnificent. For the first time in a long time, I feel in tune with my true self again.

CHAPTER SEVEN

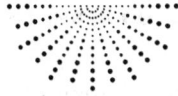

*t five o'clock in the morning on Sunday, my alarm rings, marking the inevitable end of our vacation. This last night in a hotel near the Bordeaux train station was dreadful; with a malfunctioning air conditioner and stifling heat, the temperature easily exceeded thirty-five degrees in our mosquito-infested room. Tired and saddened, I reluctantly accompany my children to the train that will take them to continue their vacation with their father.

My heart is breaking as mixed feelings battle within me. I am eager to reunite with Cam and Emily, who I missed so much during this week—but I have no desire to leave my older children. I won't see them again until September, a situation that has never happened before. Tears fall as I realize that my dream of a large, beautiful, blended family is collapsing.

Over the next few days, dark thoughts resurface, and my back begins to ache intensely again, but I don't immediately pay attention to it. After the long car journey from the Pyrenees, I decide to ease back into activity by joining the gentle morning gym group at the campsite. *I'll start with that,* I tell myself. But even this proves too much. Midway through the first session, I have to stop and ask for help to return to my spot. Tears flow as I feel angry at my failure.

Abandoning group activities, I attempt short, adapted yoga sessions in the shade of the pine trees, hoping to relax and enjoy the summer sun. But once again, I'm met with agony. Days pass, and my mind becomes increasingly fixated on the pain. *Why is my body, the same body that brought me such happiness a few weeks ago, letting me down again?*

**The body that carried her through joy and despair,
Now burdens her heart, too heavy to bear.**

August arrives, bringing a change of scenery. Camille's son Noah goes to visit his mother for the remainder of the vacation, leaving just the three of us to explore Anglet, a city I love. After departing the Bordeaux campsite in the evening, we leave our caravan at the winter storage warehouse and continue our journey south to Les Sables-d'Or.

The road is long, and my lumbar pain persists—not worse, but not better. I prop myself up with cushions and bath towels, staying awake to keep Cam company. By early morning, we arrive at Les Sables-d'Or. After a short nap in the car, we wait for our favorite bakery to open and for Emily to wake up in the backseat.

When I wake up, something feels different. My back no longer torments me; there's only a diffuse heaviness in my lower back. This minor discomfort is quickly overshadowed by the joy of rediscovering the places I love. The first few days are magical. Long walks, the beach, the sun—it all feels possible again. Everything is going well. We even indulge in an impromptu photo shoot on the Chambre d'Amour, capturing a moment of happiness under the Basque sun.

But as our return date approaches, persistent anxiety overwhelms me. The thought of going back to work, the accompanying stress, and managing family life weigh heavily on my mind. With my dark thoughts, the pain returns.

Desperate, I consult a renowned osteopath in Anglet who is highly praised online for his methods in treating lower back pain. After a few manipulations, he suggests I read *Healing Back Pain* by John E. Sarno. While he isn't able to provide much relief, his recommendation sparks hope. I immediately purchase the e-book and dive into it. Though some of Sarno's ideas have since been challenged, his emphasis on the brain's role in chronic pain resonates with me.

Buoyed by newfound hope, I push myself mentally and physically, going for a brisk walk along the promenade of Les Sables-d'Or. But after just a few meters, the pain becomes unbearable. I push harder until I can no longer put my foot on the ground. Tears stream down my face as suffering crushes me once again. Without my phone, I can't call Cam for help. Dragging myself down the street, I eventually resort to crawling. On Rue de la Falaise, passersby rush to my aid, calling for help and carrying me back to my apartment.

My morale is shattered. Once again, dark thoughts bubble to the surface: *I will never heal.*

Explaining anxiety to those who don't understand
Is like grasping at smoke with trembling hands.

Anxiety, my insidious and treacherous companion, weaves its web through my mind. It monopolizes my every thought, haunting me daily. I'm afraid of everything: the future, life itself.

As digestive problems, insomnia, and difficulty falling asleep become constant, I'm consumed by an intense sense of inferiority and uselessness. Most days, I lie in bed, participating less and less in activities with Cam and Emily. The tension in the apartment is palpable. Crushing fatigue annihilates any desire or motivation.

Adding to my despair, my left leg begins to exhibit strange symptoms: loss of sensation, electric shocks that last for hours, and complete numbness. By the end of August, I am bedridden, neglecting even my hygiene. Through the window, I watch families heading to the beach. The Miramar lighthouse, immobile and majestic, is my only silent companion.

I'm now on extremely high doses of morphine, but nothing alleviates my suffering. My sciatic pain has culminated in complete paralysis of my left leg. I also develop early signs of cauda equina syndrome, with genitourinary and sphincter dysfunction. My condition is nothing short of a slow agony.

So what's left of us?
Cam shoulders it all, torn between giving Emily a
good vacation and caring for me.

We are clearly drifting apart. I am dependent on him for everything, no longer feeling like a person, let alone a woman. Even empathy from friends and family deepens my guilt:

"Come on, pull yourself together—it'll pass!"

"Don't let yourself get down."

"You're a fighter—you'll get through this!"

Trapped in a whirlwind of negative thoughts, I dwell on my pain and its perceived unfairness. I fixate on what could have been and what should have been. My past haunts me, and my future terrifies me. Figuratively, I am going in circles. Literally, I can't even walk.

The looming drive back to Lille fills me with dread. A doctor at SOS Médecin in Biarritz urges me to return home immediately to consult my neurosurgeon. He mentions his wife, who delayed treatment for a similar condition and now faces permanent consequences. He warns me that my paralysis and cauda equina symptoms signal an urgent crisis.

CHAPTER EIGHT

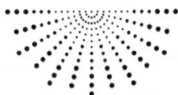

I'm back home. Finally. Two days later, Cam carries me into the waiting room of the doctor's office. The pain is so intense that I can't sit still, so I agonize between standing, sitting, kneeling, and lying on the floor—it's torture. The waiting room is full, but thankfully, the other (deeply kind) patients allow me to go ahead of them.

As we speak with the surgeon, fear creeps back in. He prescribes Solupred to ease my pain—a steroid I've tried before, with no success. If there's no improvement in ten days, surgery will be considered. I trust this doctor, but the words of the practitioner in Biarritz haunt me: *"You must be taken care of immediately, or you'll suffer lifelong consequences. Every day is crucial."*

As if one misfortune isn't enough, I catch a severe form of Covid-19. What a gift. I'm in an unimaginable state: living on a medicalized mattress on the floor in the middle of the living room, bedpan and all. I won't even describe my gastrointestinal misery. The sciatic pain adds another layer to this ordeal. My pharmacist, Charlotte, even makes house calls just for me. The last shred of my pride vanishes.

As a last resort, I'm referred to a highly reputed rehabilitation specialist at the Lille University Hospital. By sheer luck, a cancellation allows me to see her the next day. She subjects me to a battery of tests: sensitivity evaluations, motor skill assessments, and physiological analyses. Her findings are alarming, confirming the pessimistic diagnosis from Biarritz: I am losing motor function on the entire left side of my body, from my pelvis to my toes. Total paralysis is imminent.

In a panic, I call my general practitioner, who sees me within the hour. He's an old-fashioned doctor who knows his patients well. When I tell him my suffering is unbearable, he believes me. Concerned, he urgently prescribes an MRI. I will never thank him enough.

After countless phone calls and relentless perseverance, I secure an appointment the next day. Despite sedatives, I can't stay still in the machine. The pain is too much. I cry, scream, and twist, overwhelmed by an uncontrollable panic attack. A nurse holds my hand as my tears turn into sobs. Thankfully, though blurry, the MRI results are clear— and devastating. The radiologist intervenes directly with my neurosurgeon to ensure I'm seen immediately.

The next day, my neurosurgeon reviews my case. His concern is evident. My condition has rapidly deteriorated, threatening my motor abilities entirely. After a year and a half of daily suffering and countless medical dead ends, the truth is undeniable: my L5-S1 hernia has ruptured. The guillotine has fallen.

A crisis decision is made: I will undergo surgery the next morning —Sunday, September 11, at 8:00 a.m. That same day, I'm admitted to the hospital. It's the longest night of my life.

Cam tries to support me over text, but when he goes to bed, I feel utterly alone. I scream in pain, my cries echoing through the hospital floor. Sleep is impossible; the agony relentless. Nurses come to check on me throughout the night. Some are kind and try to reassure me; others brusquely tell me I'm disturbing the other patients.

I beg for something to help me sleep, but they say only a doctor can authorize an increased dose. Hours later, an irritated doctor finally arrives, gives me a strong sedative via a drip, and leaves. Slowly, my body succumbs to exhaustion, and I drift off.

* * *

At 6:00 a.m., groggy but awake, I'm prepared for the operating room. Everything moves quickly. The surgeon greets me warmly and reassures me: *"In a few hours, this will be nothing more than a bad memory."* Before I can process his words, the anesthesia takes hold.

When I wake, it's over. The surgery is done. The doctor is satisfied with the structural success of the operation. However, my left leg remains paralyzed for now.

I stay in the hospital for the next three days as the doctors monitor my recovery, particularly my urinary functions, to ensure I don't need a catheter. Though somewhat relieved, I am far from whole.

PART II
MY WINTER WILL BE STUDIOUS

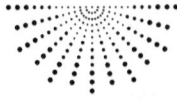

Walking in the sleet, when your body feels so weak,
And the sadness in your eyes, you can no longer
    disguise.

Don't give up, don't look back,
Straighten up, keep on track, and just keep
    pushin' on.
Although it's hard on the way, your heart and soul
    are strong.

And the cloudy sky has a silver lining—
That's the reason why you get up every morning.
Nothing else, nothing more, doesn't matter where you
    turn.
You live and learn.

If you're feeling down, liquor leads to a place
    unknown,
And your dreams are put on hold
As you watch your life unfold.

Don't give up, don't look back,
Straighten up, keep on track, and just keep
pushin' on.
Although it's hard on the way, your heart and soul
are strong.

And the cloudy sky has a silver lining—
That's the reason why you get up every morning.
Nothing else, nothing more, doesn't matter where you
turn.
You live and learn, just live and learn.

There's no reason to complain,
You have to stand strong and embrace the pain.
And only you know what you have to do,
'Cause there's no one—no one—who'll do it for you.

You live and learn, just live and learn…

CHAPTER NINE

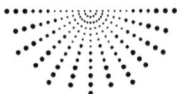

J wake up groggy. The first blow to my morale comes just days after the operation. Messages of affection pour in. Everyone seems thrilled for me. Of course, they assume that now, after surgery, I'm finally relieved and free from back pain. Why wouldn't they?

But that assumption is false—and deeply frustrating.

I wasn't operated on for back pain; I was operated on for *cauda equina syndrome* and paralysis in my left leg. As a result, the surgeon partially saved my left leg, but my foot remains paralyzed, and I suffer from severe neuropathic pain. The worst part of it all?

I still have back pain.

I *still* have back pain.

It's hard to bounce back. My feelings, like my morale, are on a relentless roller coaster, oscillating between sciatic pain, neuropathic pain, and this persistent back pain—the origin of which remains unknown. Withdrawing from my medications adds another layer of misery, bringing tremors, cold sweats, insomnia, dizziness, and a host of uncomfortable sensations.

To help me cope, a dedicated team of psychologists, psychiatrists, and nurses from the medico-psychological center takes turns visiting my home daily. Their support helps me break free from the vicious cycle of depression and suicidal thoughts. They even leave their mobile numbers with Cam so he can call them at any hour if an emergency arises.

It's October. I've always loved the flamboyant colors of autumn—the smell of freshly fallen leaves, the wind rustling through the trees. What a joy it once was to go chestnut hunting with my little one, gathering colorful leaves to decorate the table for Mummy's and Daddy's birthdays.

But this year, there's no celebration in sight. My heart feels like it's stuck in winter, wholly dormant.

After six weeks of required healing, I'm finally allowed to stand for longer periods. My physiotherapist begins visiting three times a week for mobilization exercises. During my postoperative check-up, the surgeon declares the operation a success. He explains with satisfaction that the nerve conflict problem has been resolved.

"As for the rest," he adds, "you narrowly escaped a worse fate. You should consider yourself lucky to walk without much limping."

As for the residual pains? *Learn to live with them.*

I sigh. Nothing I haven't heard before.

The neuropathic pains make sense to me—they're the direct consequence of the nerve damage caused by the herniated disc and its rupture. The compression of my sciatic nerve and its roots created dysfunction in both my peripheral and central nervous systems. Even though the nerve is no longer compressed, it has been irreparably damaged.

But what about my other pains? These persistent lower back pains, which supposedly no longer have any structural cause? I feel like I'm back to square one, stuck with standard pain management strategies that ask me to resign myself to a life of suffering. But I don't want to live like this. I want to *heal*. I refuse to accept what is happening—what is *still* happening.

I begin to notice contradictions in what health professionals have told me. If my back pain is caused by structural degeneration, as they claim, why am I not in pain *all the time*? Some mornings, I feel noticeably better. My physiotherapy sessions are sometimes nearly painless, yet other days, I struggle to even sit upright.

Two weeks ago, every breath felt like a metal bar stabbing through my back, paired with searing pain in my leg. But recently, I've resumed yoga, and my pain has eased significantly. Yet today, the pain is back. The night was unbearable, and I'm dwelling on family troubles again.

I've always tried to reconcile everyone's expectations, avoid conflicts, and ease tensions. Preserving this precarious balance at all costs has finally backfired—and I'm paying the price.

Are my pains influenced by my emotional state? Perhaps by fatigue?

Yes.

When I'm filled with positive thoughts and inspired by projects, my pains noticeably fade. It's glaring. I begin to understand that the truth must lie elsewhere.

I commit to exploring more deeply the link between my chronic pain and my state of mind—in other words, the powerful connection between body and mind.

CHAPTER TEN

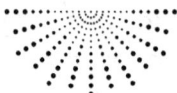

I embark on an international quest for answers. I need references, mentors, and certainties. My journey begins in the United States, where I delve deeply into the works of Professor John E. Sarno. His books, which I had briefly browsed last summer, now take on profound significance. I discover that mind–body medicine is far from a novel concept. As I read through his pages, I immediately recognize myself—and it's a revelation! Finally, I have a reason why, despite a successful surgery and a "healed" back, I still experience these damn stabbing pains, sometimes even more intense than before the operation.

When life, pain, and sorrow intertwine,
Salvation whispers, a light to shine.
This sadness does not have to be mine.

Questions of existence, answers to find,
Yearning for truth defined.
Longing for hope in life, a reason to feel fine—
Waiting for, waiting for, waiting for what?

Clutching at signs and fate's gentle sway,
Miracles, dreams, or the price to pay.
Suffering echoing, day by day—
Waiting for, waiting for, waiting for what?

In the seventeenth century, Western medicine took a decisive turn: no longer would patients be treated holistically, as ancient practices did, by analyzing the mind and body as inseparable entities. Instead, the body became viewed as a machine, its parts replaceable through modern medicine, while the mind was treated as a separate entity, disconnected from the physical body.

This shift enabled rapid progress in surgery and pharmaceuticals, but it also introduced limitations. John E. Sarno, a professor of orthopedic medicine and rehabilitation at New York University, re-examined the connection between the mind and body. He studied how emotional and spiritual life influences physical ailments.

In his patients, Sarno observed chronic pain, gastrointestinal issues, dermatological disorders, and generalized pain with no detectable structural causes. When traditional treatments failed to provide relief, he introduced a new perspective: *tension myositis syndrome (TMS)*.

At first, I wonder if Sarno is some kind of quack or guru, preaching pseudoscience without real evidence. But as I dig deeper, I find he is a highly respected physician who has helped liberate thousands of people from chronic pain, either directly or through professionals trained in his methods.

I then discover Dr. Howard Schubiner, founder of the Mind–Body Medicine Program. Available and attentive, he takes the time to converse with me and, more importantly, to enlighten me. Later, I'll have the privilege of exchanging ideas with him during the development of my own mind–body connection method.

In his book *Unlearn Your Pain*, Dr. Schubiner explains: "Just as the nervous system has learned to experience pain, it can learn to be free from pain." By building on Sarno's work, Schubiner empowers individuals to become active participants in their healing process, breaking free from sole dependence on doctors and medications.

He writes of witnessing "miracles that are not miracles at all" every day. Patients, after years of suffering and medical wandering, free themselves from chronic pain by uncovering its deep-seated causes.

This awareness revives my hopes of one day living normally again —of putting on my socks by myself, playing with my little one, and going on Sunday morning runs. It rekindles my dreams of bigger things, too: running the New York Marathon, visiting my best friend in Arizona, surfing with my family in San Diego, and making music again.

My quest for truth, supported by Cam's unwavering encouragement, gives us a new challenge to face together. We turn toward the future with renewed hope, ready to ride this new wave of discovery and healing.

CHAPTER ELEVEN

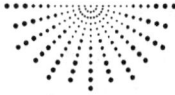

At the end of 2022, my quest for answers takes me to Australia, where I have the honor of participating in a clinical trial at the prestigious eCentreClinic at Macquarie University in Sydney. It is a true blessing to be admitted into such a comprehensive e-learning experimental protocol.

1. My Pain Is Real

Since ancient times, physicians have discussed the psychological aspect of pain. Despite this, twentieth-century medicine adopted a linear approach: imaging is performed, lesions are analyzed, and treatments are based on the assumption that the intensity and characteristics of pain directly reflect the type and extent of the lesions.

Thankfully, in recent years, the definition of pain has evolved to include its biopsychological dimension. Pain is now understood as a physiological process where the brain generates a pain signal in response to a perceived threat, whether physical or psychological.

Unfortunately, treatments have been slow to integrate this understanding. In the absence of a clearly identifiable structural cause, I've been told countless times that my pain is "in my head," as if I have full control over my experience. My pain is *not* in my head—even if it is generated by my brain.

Ninety-eight percent of headache-related pains are non-structural, caused by the brain; the same is true for 99% of fibromyalgia pain, 99% of irritable bowel syndrome pain, 90% of pelvic pain, and 85% of back or neck pain. The statistics speak for themselves.

2. My Knowledge Is My Power

The therapeutic education portion of the Australian program takes me back to my neuroscience studies at the Free Faculty of Medicine. Now, the word *pain* has a deeper meaning for me. I truly know what it means to hurt.

Therapeutic education is a scientifically recognized treatment. The more I understand what is happening in my brain and body, the easier it becomes to restore "zero pain" neural connections by reducing fear and, consequently, painful symptoms.

3. The Brain Decides Everything

When my neighbor's alarm goes off at 2:00 a.m., I can't ignore it—it does its job perfectly. Similarly, pain is the brain's alarm system. When the brain detects a threat, it triggers pain to protect the body.

I recall a trail run on the Côte d'Opale a few years ago, where I stepped into a hole and sprained my ankle. Nociceptors in my foot, stimulated by the pressure, sent an electrical signal via my nerves to my brain. This signal, called nociception, is not a pain message but a primitive warning of potential harm.

Upon receiving the signal, my brain analyzed my emotional state, previous painful experiences, and overall health to decide on the most appropriate response: flight, fight, tears, and/or pain. All this happened in an instant. The pain I felt was created in my brain, not my foot. My brain, based on its programming, decided how much pain I should feel.

. . .

4. Pain Is Sometimes Beneficial

I was frustrated not to finish the race, despite my training. But in hindsight, I should have been grateful: continuing to run would have worsened my injury, delayed healing, and extended my recovery time. When my ankle healed, the pain disappeared, allowing me to gradually resume activity.

5. Pain Is a Normal Physiological Response

When we face a threat, our body reacts with three options: fight, flight, or freeze. These survival mechanisms, conceptualized by physiologist W. Cannon in the 1920s, enable us to cope with danger.

Whether the threat is physical (a lion or a hot pan) or psychological (trauma or stress), the body secretes adrenaline and cortisol, signaling the brain that immediate action is needed. The brain enters alert mode, heightening our senses. Once the threat passes, it takes 6–20 minutes for the body to return to its calm state.

6. Pain Is Influenced by the Biopsychosocial Context

Pain is deeply personal and subjective, shaped by our biology, psychology, and social context. The brain activates areas responsible for sensations, movements, emotions, and memory simultaneously, making each person's experience unique.

Like a computer, the brain creates programs based on past experiences and filters environmental signals: *Have I received this signal before? What were the consequences? What is the context?* These filters influence how the brain interprets danger and whether it generates pain.

7. Thoughts Shape Emotions, and Emotions Shape Actions

Our thoughts, whether conscious or unconscious, drive our emotions, which in turn influence our actions. The brain relies on this programming to decide whether or not to generate pain. Factors like anxiety, fears, beliefs, personality traits, and adaptability all play a role.

Pain reflects not just a biological issue but a combination of everything happening in the body, mind, and environment.

8. I Am Not Fragile

The anomalies and degenerations in my body are like internal "wrinkles" or "gray hairs." They are normal. As the late Professor Sarno put it, they are "normal abnormalities."

I have the right to run, jump, practice yoga, and carry my daughter. Resuming physical activities gradually is not just possible—it's essential for my healing.

9. Pain Is Not My Enemy

Pain is the body's alarm system, prompting action to address a potential threat. It's a vital response, developed over millennia to help our ancestors survive in hostile environments.

The conclusion is clear: I must not ignore my brain's warnings. Instead, I must strive to understand its message.

This program and its insights rekindle my hope. With Cam's unwavering support, I look to the future with renewed determination. Together, we face this next challenge head-on, ready to embrace the opportunities that come with understanding and healing.

CHAPTER TWELVE

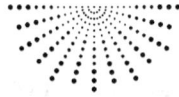

*T*he therapeutic education program now tackles the final secrets of pain: it's not just hungry lions that make my brain roar. Now that I understand the mechanisms and causes of pain, I must dive deeper to uncover why my pain has become chronic.

Truth #1: Pain Is an Opinion, Not a Fact

Pain is the brain's *opinion* in response to a real or perceived threat —not an absolute fact. As Professor Sarno brilliantly highlighted, pain can have psychoanalytic causes. The brain stages very real psychosomatic pains, a term that, though often stigmatized, represents genuine suffering for those who endure it. I am here to testify to its reality.

According to Sarno, the brain creates pain to divert attention from deep emotional issues. The brain determines that we lack the immediate resources to confront this psychological suffering and offers us physical pain instead—an "uncomfortable comfort" it deems more bearable than the emotional turmoil it perceives as unmanageable.

Other scientists suggest that pain emerges when the brain can no longer repress emotions. Pain becomes the brain's plea for us to care for ourselves, forgive ourselves, and express our needs.

Regardless of the theory, it is a self-defense mechanism—our body's response to a perceived unconscious danger. The brain believes this threat could compromise our survival and, in extreme cases, lead to self-destruction. When we confront the real causes of our pain, the symptoms often disappear because the pain is no longer needed to protect us.

To heal, I must address the psychological origins of my pain, not just its physical manifestations.

Truth #2: Hypersensitive = Hyper-Painful

Chronic pain, now recognized as a disease in its own right, is like a dysfunctional alarm system—a brain perpetually in alert mode and a hypersensitive nervous system. Unfortunately, this heightened state doesn't always reflect reality.

Sometimes the brain makes mistakes. When it constantly detects threats, it concludes that the body is in constant danger. This overactivation overwhelms the brain with incessant danger signals it can no longer inhibit. Nervous hypersensitivity sets in, and pain becomes unpredictable.

One day, I'm in severe pain; the next, it's significantly reduced. Some Sundays, I can play with my daughter all afternoon, even though that very morning I couldn't get out of bed.

Acute pain activates the brain's emergency systems for short periods. Chronic pain, however, keeps these systems on indefinitely. Prolonged activation leads to high cortisol levels, the stress hormone, causing generalized distress and exacerbating chronic pain. This persistent state of hypersensitivity hinders healing.

Our bodies, like finely tuned machines, rely on homeostasis—a balance of systems. But when hypersensitivity takes over, the balance is lost, and all systems overreact.

Truth #3: The Brain Forgets Nothing

Vitiant artus aegra contagia mentis. In Latin, this means, "The contagious diseases of the soul affect the limbs" (Ovid, *Tristia*).

As someone who studied Latin as a living language, I can't resist quoting Ovid, who understood centuries ago that pain can blur the lines between mind and body.

In more than 50% of cases, pain has both physical and psychological origins. Pain can persist for years simply because it has been recorded somewhere in the labyrinth of our memory.

We cannot erase it—but we can tame it and learn to coexist with it.

Truth #4: Hypersensitive = Hyper-Conditioned

The "fight or flight" response, essential for human survival, is a powerful asset. Our brain learns specific patterns of response to protect us, refining them over a lifetime of experiences.

This is where Pavlov's famous experiments with his dog come into play. When Ivan Pavlov rang a bell and presented food, the dog salivated. After repeating this process, Pavlov rang the bell without offering food, and the dog still salivated.

This same conditioning process triggers my pain. My brain generates a conditioned response to harmless stimuli—like leaning forward or even thinking about pain. A simple, innocuous movement becomes linked to danger, causing my hypersensitive brain to sound the alarm unnecessarily.

A New Understanding

Through this program, I'm learning that my pain is not an enemy but a misunderstood signal. By reframing my relationship with it, I hope to break free from these conditioned responses and reclaim the balance that chronic pain has stolen from me.

PART III
MY SPRING FINALLY ARRIVES

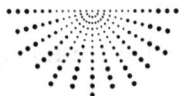

Every story has its tale but may leave you unaware,
Like a boat without a sail, trying hard to get
somewhere.

Never ask the reason why it comes and goes or
passes by—
It's just a song, a simple rhyme, that takes you through
the winds of time.

Les ruisseaux font les grandes rivières.

And the pass, pass, pass, passing time, time, time
carries on every day,
And you will see, see, see in the sign, the way.

And the pass, pass, pass, passing time, time, time takes
you on anyway,
You will see, see, see in the fine, the way.

If the melody is good and the lyrics understood,

It could mean something you despise or bring tears to
your eyes.

There's no need to underline if you can read between
the lines—
Something you have never heard, a few old chords and
simple words.

Les ruisseaux font les grandes rivières.

And the pass, pass, pass, passing time, time, time
carries on every day,
And you will see, see, see in the sign, the way.

And the pass, pass, pass, passing time, time, time takes
you on anyway,
You will see, see, see in the fine, the way.

An old guitar that's out of tune, an empty page, an
empty den,
Sitting in this lonely room with just my passion and
a pen.

Les ruisseaux font les grandes rivières.

CHAPTER THIRTEEN

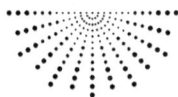

Tomorrow Begins Today

I decide to definitively turn away from studying pain and its mechanisms, choosing instead to wholeheartedly embrace the construction of my pain-free future. This new chapter will focus on integrating the emotional component of my suffering into my self-therapy.

Healing from a mind–body syndrome requires adopting a psychological approach rather than a purely structural one. Thinking psychologically means confronting everything that consumes me from within: resentment, anger, sadness—perhaps even hatred. Who knows what discoveries await in the depths of my unconscious as I embark on this introspection, this psychological investigation?

Now that I have the necessary knowledge and skills, I feel ready to tackle the psychological roots of my pain, guided by Professor Sarno's equation:

Chronic pain = one third adverse childhood experiences + one third daily stress + one third predisposing personality traits.

The toolbox of the mind–body connection method is abundant and diverse. I have explored many tools, and this very diversity enriches the approach. There is no single path to healing chronic pain. What is certain, however, is the necessity of observing what is happening in our minds in order to adequately address what is happening in our bodies.

CHAPTER FOURTEEN

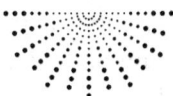

*J*t's January 2023. It's been more than three months since my surgery. The myriad of programs I have explored until this point have brought significant functional improvements, but none has provided me with complete healing. I still experience pain, and so I have no intention of giving up.

Injustice felt, never causing harm's strife,
Yet fear echoes loud in the corridors of my life.

I'm now focused on the common denominator among the various mind–body therapies I've followed: the fear factor. Until now, I believed my number one enemy was pain. However, from this day forward, I will no longer mistake my number one enemy: that enemy is fear, eating me from within. For months, no one has managed to relieve my back pain, and all attempts to treat its symptoms have ended in dismal failure. And it's all because the problem is not of structural nature but rather stems from my nervous system being chronically on high alert. My fearful brain overprotects me and goes into survival mode. Like an excessively protective parent, my brain prevents me from fully living.

In reality, my pains are in no way inexplicable. They are the result of thousands of years of evolution that led to an extreme sophistication of my "super" brain. In my case, three fears combine. Most of the time, I am still immersed in deep depression, a prisoner of my rumination, negative anticipations, and sometimes suicidal thoughts. Then, the fear of a recurrence always lingers in the back of my mind. I spend a lot of time in Facebook groups where, reading posts, I get the impression that all back surgery patients face recurrences. Thus, I am terrified at the thought that it might happen to me, too. Finally, after months of excruciating pain, my brain has learned to be in pain and is stuck in a fear-and-pain spiral from which it cannot escape.

Psychologist Robert Merton was the first to identify the phenomenon of self-fulfilling prophecies. When one is convinced that an event will happen, this event is more likely to occur. One holding such a belief unconsciously generates behaviors and emotions that make the event more likely to happen. Thus, I clearly realize that the fears tormenting me fuel my pains. I remember my last brisk walk in Anglet, which ended in crawling in the street, ashamed and helpless, trying desperately to get back to my apartment. Everything seems so obvious now! Reading the book by Professor Sarno diagonally was one thing, but putting it into practice was another. Even if I could discern the potential psychological causes of my pain, I had not yet begun to explore my problems and had not taken any steps to solve them. So, my brain simply made me understand: "Not so fast—I'm still afraid, and I think I'm still in danger!" In reality, anxiety was eating away at me from the inside and preventing me from moving forward—literally and figuratively.

CHAPTER FIFTEEN

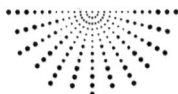

On Sunday, February 5, 2023, nearly 550 people gathered for a candlelight vigil in memory of Lucas, a thirteen-year-old boy who took his own life after enduring years of bullying at school. This tragic event hit me deeply. I, too, was hindered by school bullying. It led me into anorexia and forced my parents to withdraw me from school. The mere thought of stepping onto school grounds terrified me, isolating me completely.

I've always had a tumultuous relationship with school. Though I love learning and have an insatiable thirst for knowledge, I've never felt at home in a school environment. Even as a child, I struggled to find acceptance among my peers—or even among teachers, who often criticized me.

"Since you've finished all your work, you could at least be kind and help your classmates."

Those words still echo in my mind, even thirty years later. They left me with a lasting fear of never doing enough for others and a sense of guilt whenever I take time for myself.

When I entered middle school, my parents and I chose what we thought was a good institution—one where I hoped to find support and belonging. Yet middle school, that turbulent time of self-discovery and conflict, proved unkind to me. Torn between blending into a group and forging my own path, I felt out of sync with my peers.

I didn't share their interests and had only a few friends. I became "weird," "nerd," "pimply glasses girl," and "Miss Know-It-All."

One day during gym class, a group of popular girls decided to target me. When the lifeguard and teachers weren't looking, they grabbed me and held my head underwater. I flailed and gasped, feeling like I might drown. Though it probably lasted only seconds, it felt like forever. The trauma lingered.

What did they gain by doing this? I still wonder. At the time, I would've done anything—*anything*—to make them leave me alone.

This was just one incident in a long series of torments. My glasses were stolen and hidden. I was locked in bathroom stalls. They put dissected frog remains in my pencil case, tore up my notebooks, and left cruel notes in my backpack. They told me I didn't belong.

No one defended me—not that I blame them. Anyone who sided with me would likely suffer the same torment. One day, pushed to the brink, I burst into tears in the middle of the courtyard, surrounded by my tormentors.

In those years, I played tennis and even won tournaments. On the surface, I was a cheerful pre-teen. But darkness crept in. I began skipping meals, hiding unfinished food, and letting my Yorkshire terrier, Lipton, clean my plate. I hid my weight loss under baggy clothes.

During anxiety attacks, I retreated to the bathroom to vomit. Strangely, this self-destructive behavior gave me a sense of power. The less I ate, the more energized I felt. It was as if I had superpowers. My tennis improved, my learning quickened, and I felt invincible—until the euphoria gave way to emptiness.

As my weight plummeted below 36 kilos, the physical toll became undeniable. Pain radiated through my body, rendering my right side almost useless. I had to relearn to write with my left hand and give up tennis altogether. Yet even the prospect of hospitalization didn't faze me.

Thankfully, my parents refused to give up on me. They pulled me out of school and supported me as best they could, though they, too, felt helpless. At home, I spent my days singing—my only escape from the overwhelming emptiness. Singing was the one thing that made me feel alive.

* * *

The turning point came when I traveled to England, where my host family introduced me to pub performances. Behind a microphone, I found a place I belonged. The positive emotions I experienced on stage helped me begin to eat again.

Back home, though, I faced a terrifying wake-up call. One night, I fainted in my sleep. Disoriented, I stumbled out of bed, only to collapse. Lipton barked to alert my parents, but in my fall, I landed on him. He had saved me, but I couldn't save him.

This chapter of my life, one I've never openly shared before now, is deeply tied to my chronic pain. Bullying left scars—not just emotional ones, but physical manifestations in my body. Studies show that bullied children are significantly more likely to consider suicide and may later endure chronic pain because of their experiences.

As a teenager, my brain cut off hunger as an alarm signal. It took me years to rediscover that sensation. With time, the support of my parents, and the Rotary Club, I left the toxic school environment for Canada, where I slowly rebuilt my confidence.

I realized that if I could "turn off" hunger back then, I could now "turn off" pain when it is no longer necessary for my survival.

* * *

Oscar Wilde once said,
"The best way to resist temptation is to yield to it."

I believe the same is true for pain. When I stopped fighting it in a fierce, unequal battle, like David against Goliath, I could finally confront the messages my brain was trying to convey.

This realization changed my life. To heal, I must reprogram my brain, addressing its fear of perceived dangers—whether physical or psychological. By reframing pain as an error in my brain's programming, I can reduce its grip. By confronting buried truths and exploring long-held fears, I will free myself from their hold and open new doors to the future.

The essence of a thousand things,
Verses or prose, the melody sings.
Have a wise soul, where wisdom springs.

Way beyond …
Beyond the steps in the night,
Beyond the voice's tremor slight,
Beyond shadows in a heart,
Beyond the sins we're trying to fight.

I have not said my last word. I will defeat this Goliath.

CHAPTER SIXTEEN

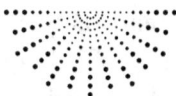

*T*oday, a Boost of Motivation!

It's all about programming. The brain, with its billions of neurons interacting through intricate neural pathways, is a dynamic and adaptive organ. Neuroplasticity—the brain's ability to modify and reorganize neural connections based on experience—is a cornerstone of my healing journey. Over time, neural pathways that are rarely used weaken, while frequently used ones strengthen. The more a thought resides in our brain and elicits emotions, the more efficient the neural pathway becomes. Brain plasticity is a significant asset in my recovery because it means I can reprogram my brain. I have the power to help it regain optimal functioning.

To study brain plasticity, researchers often conduct brain scans on women before, during, and after pregnancy. Their findings? A mother's brain undergoes structural and functional changes, developing increased vigilance to threats in the environment to protect her baby. This transformation explains the seemingly uncanny phenomenon that compels me to wake up just a few minutes before my little one every day.

The brain is constantly learning, perpetually evolving. When we learn to play the piano, surf, or knit, new neural pathways form. A remarkable example of brain plasticity is learning to swim. It's not about consciously activating leg and arm muscles—it's about integrating a complex cognitive and muscular activity. Neural pathways form seamlessly, without conscious effort. Unfortunately, the brain makes no distinction between positive learning (like swimming) and negative experiences, such as chronic pain.

Pain neural pathways develop from a combination of factors, including stressful events, repressed emotions, and self-imposed pressures. Anxiety, self-criticism, and daily stressors are my primary triggers. The more I hurt, the more my brain learns to hurt, reinforcing pain pathways. Over time, these pathways become a sort of neural highway of pain—a pattern my brain has almost become addicted to. But there's hope: since these connections are learned, they can also be unlearned.

At the L'Espoir Center in Villeneuve-d'Ascq, I found a profound example of this as an art therapist. The center treats patients who have undergone amputations, many of whom experience phantom limb pain. In such cases, the brain's mental map of the body is outdated, and therapy focuses on restoring new physical, motor, and sensory awareness. While not universally effective, the widespread success of this therapy highlights the incredible plasticity of the brain and its ability to retrace pain-free neural pathways. Inspired by this, I've integrated similar techniques into my rehabilitation at home for my left leg and foot. Though progress is gradual, I've observed notable positive effects, including a significant reduction in the burning sensations that have plagued me for so long.

The brain's adaptability is my ally. Just as it can learn pain, it can unlearn it. With time, effort, and focus, I am forging a new path—one that leads to freedom from chronic pain.

CHAPTER SEVENTEEN

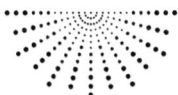

*M*y story boils down to a slew of broken connections. With each fruitless consultation, my confidence in medicine weakens. Cam's doubts about my ability to heal grow more evident, and together, our certainty in finding a solution dwindles day by day. Enthusiastic remarks have gradually been replaced by resigned comments and serious considerations of adaptation rather than recovery. I remain desperate, with aimlessness sowing confusion, doubt, and fear within me—and where there is fear, there is pain.

To move forward, it's crucial that I regain confidence in myself and my future. Often in life, we are our own solutions. Feeling assured that surgery and medication cannot address my neuroplastic pain, I must delve deeper into the mind–body connection. This unity between the mind and body forms the foundation of my MBC (Mind–Body Connection) method. My brain has lost its privileged connection with my body, and the challenge now is to restore this link by addressing both holistically. The key lies in fully understanding the emotional component of pain.

My chronic pain is a complex concoction influenced by past trauma, daily stress, limiting beliefs, negative thoughts, a hostile environment, poor sleep, an unbalanced diet, and a sedentary lifestyle. My job now is to create a healing method that addresses each ingredient. I feel a mix of excitement, apprehension, and fear. This new approach is my last hope, requiring patience and perseverance to nourish my mind, body, and soul. It's a leap into the unknown—but what if it works? And how can I share what I learn with others who suffer like me?

My brain must first unlearn its bad habits. I must tackle the emotional roots of fear—repression, catastrophization—and the fear of physical movement, or kinesiophobia. Replacing these fears with new interpretations of daily signals will reprogram my brain and restore its balance.

To heal, I will draw daily from the MBC toolbox:
1. **Express my emotions authentically**
2. **Reprogram my brain away from fear**
3. **Calm my nervous system**

To achieve this, I will follow the three L's: *learning* more about myself, *living* fully in my emotions, and *launching* my action plan. I will stop waiting for miracles, new medications, or surgical interventions. Instead, I will reshape my life to retrain my brain and build new, pain-free neural pathways. I will become my own therapy by engaging in active strategies to heal and move freely again.

To reprogram my brain, I'll employ the ELCAF tool:
Express, Liberate, Calm, Accept, and Flourish.

Expressing my emotions is essential for freeing myself from their influence. The body isn't just a machine with malfunctioning parts—it's far more complex. Living pain-free means understanding chronic pain through a biopsychosocial lens rather than simply a physical or biological one. Putting words to my pain will allow me to release it, step by step.

With enthusiasm, motivation, and patience, I will challenge old certainties and unearth buried truths. My perception of the world and my lifestyle will need to evolve. By understanding my limits, I will learn to work with them rather than against them. Like a conductor harmonizing an orchestra, I will coordinate every element of my life to enjoy it fully—without burning the candle at both ends.

Calming my nervous system will become a daily routine. Techniques such as meditation, pranayama, yoga, self-hypnosis, and visualization will help me handle life's challenges more effectively. Relaxing doesn't mean "doing nothing"; it's about accumulating the resources I need to thrive. Slowing down won't mean less activity, but rather doing more with less stress while rediscovering life's pleasures.

By abandoning automatic negative thoughts and adopting constructive behaviors, I can progressively reprogram my brain. I will block neural pathways of fear and pain, exploring instead those of joy, gratitude, and happiness. I will accept my brain's alerts as mere signals —not as threats—and embrace my emotions as natural and fleeting. I am the protagonist of my life, and I will celebrate every victory, no matter how small. By anchoring myself in the present, I will let go of the past and stop anticipating the future with pessimism.

Finally, I will choose my best future. No longer will unspoken thoughts, indecision, or inaction dictate my path. This may require difficult decisions: distancing myself from toxic influences, making peace with past traumas, or accepting that not everything unfolds as I wish. Though challenging, I trust in my courage and determination to guide me toward a life of freedom from pain.

I will create my own Swiss army knife of healing—an arsenal of tools and techniques to manage emotions and regain physical movement. Each piece is essential to my full recovery.

Embarking on this journey of healing, I acknowledge that the storm may rage at times. In those moments, I will remember to do less and *be* more. After a lifetime of rushing from one project to another, I will embrace stillness and rediscover life's small pleasures. Like a gardener preparing the soil, I will cultivate the fertile ground necessary for healing.

Acceptance is the final stage of my journey—not just acceptance, but acceptance intertwined with resilience. Through the mind–body connection, I am gradually reconnecting with hope. The pain has not disappeared, but its presence no longer consumes me. By learning to express my needs and emotions, I am opening myself to the world once more, envisioning a happy and fulfilling future.

The discovery of mind–body medicine has allowed me to rebuild emotional resilience, and with it, I will reshape my life. Pain may have been a part of my story, but it will not define its ending.

CHAPTER EIGHTEEN

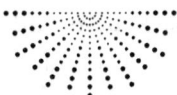

*U*ntil now, my quest for answers had been limited to the A-side of my life's record, a sorrowful lament of chronic suffering and fruitless searches for structural solutions. It was the story I recounted countless times during my medical wanderings. But true healing lies on the B-side—a side that reveals the deep-seated causes of my pain, where the unspoken truths and hidden connections finally come to light.

Looking back, three troubling aspects of my pain stand out: its symptoms appear and vanish suddenly; exhaustive medical examinations reveal no structural cause; and my pain always coincides with trauma or significant stress. With hindsight, these connections now seem glaringly obvious. Equipped with newfound clarity, I am piecing together the puzzle of my symptoms and the triggering events that shaped them.

The origins of my pain trace back to adolescence, where the shadow of bullying disrupted an otherwise happy childhood. The torment led to repeated tendinitis, a disabling tennis elbow, and the consuming grip of anorexia. Later, a sudden shoulder pain haunted me for months after learning of my grandmother's unexpected passing. Her death during a routine operation left me feeling blindsided and betrayed. The guilt of not being there for her and the anger at being kept in the dark overwhelmed me. No medical examination could find anything wrong with my shoulder, yet the pain persisted for months—until, just as inexplicably, it disappeared.

Migraines soon became unwelcome visitors, peaking during my demanding career as a buyer and occasionally during my "on the road" artist years. Sore throats, recurrent voicelessness during performances, and tendinitis plagued me when stress mounted. And then came the final blow: chronic lower back pain and hyperalgic sciatica, pinning me to my bed and robbing me of mobility. My passion for neuroscience and art therapy—and my own history—revealed the truth: my brain has been orchestrating this symphony of pain all along. My trauma was the composer.

Early on, I believed art could heal psychological wounds. As a victim of bullying, singing, writing poems, and scribbling in my diary became lifelines. Those moments of expression were tiny bursts of happiness in a dark tunnel. My diaries, filled with raw emotion, were a totem of my resilience and a testament to writing's healing power. Over time, my writing evolved into songwriting, but giving up my artistic career in 2015 left me adrift. I felt like a bird with broken wings. My close friend Justine, who had supported me for years, urged me to seek professional help, even if it meant our friendship depended on it.

I once believed my body was invincible, capable of weathering any storm. I now know how wrong I was. This realization inspired me to incorporate expressive writing workshops into my mind–body connection method. Writing, I've found, is a powerful tool for releasing emotions and processing trauma—a way to empty the overflowing glass of feelings.

As a teenager, writing was my catharsis, my lifeline. Through the pages of my diary, I could confront my fears, frustrations, and anger without restraint or judgment. It gave meaning to my experiences and allowed me to keep moving forward. Post-bullying, my parents homeschooled me until I gradually reintegrated into high school. Those years, though challenging, were transformative. Music became my refuge, and I explored poetry, detective novels, and songwriting. My world expanded when my French teacher encouraged me to participate in a Rotary Club eloquence contest. Despite my initial resistance, I reached the finals. On the day of the competition, I stood out by integrating a rendition of *The Businessman's Blues* from *Starmania*. The experience opened unexpected doors, leading to a short exchange program in Canada and, later, a year-long cultural exchange.

In Canada, I flourished. Performing, writing, and immersing myself in artistic studies reignited my passion for life. I broke free from anorexia's grip, made lifelong friends, and filled my diaries with Polaroids, tickets, and mementos of joy. These experiences reaffirmed the transformative power of expression and connection.

Today, as I integrate expressive writing into my healing journey, I equip myself with a life journal, a pen, highlighters, and draft paper. My sanctuary is a quiet, undisturbed space where I can freely explore my emotions. For twenty to thirty minutes daily, I write without worrying about grammar or structure, letting my thoughts flow spontaneously. Music, too, has become an integral part of these sessions, with playlists ranging from Sia to AC/DC, each melody tied to a significant chapter of my life.

This practice isn't just about writing; it's about liberation. It's a chance to release pent-up emotions and reframe my experiences. Like a pencil sketching territories once thought unreachable, or a pen darkening the pages of truth, writing continues to be my compass. Through it, I'm not just documenting my journey—I'm rewriting my story.

CHAPTER NINETEEN

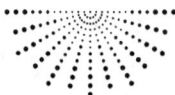

*M*y family cocoon, once my refuge and source of rejuvenation, has turned into a wellspring of stress, sadness, and anger. I am caught in a frenzied dance, no longer living—merely surviving. Just as the brain reacts to sensations like hunger, cold, and fatigue, it also responds to trauma. These traumas leave scars on the nervous system—indelible imprints, a body memory that persists even when the mind tries to forget. Over the years, my traumas remained buried, latent, waiting for me to confront them. In the meantime, neural pathways associated with fear and pain gradually overshadowed my healthier pathways. Small, fleeting pains prepared fertile ground for the eventual emergence of chronic pain.

Recent family trauma rekindled the feelings of anger and injustice I experienced as a child, leaving me grappling with alexithymia—a profound difficulty in expressing my emotions or putting words to them. Naturally joyful and talkative, I now find myself walled in sadness and enveloped in unusual silence. I feel detached from the world, as if observing my life from outside myself. When my little one innocently asks, "Is your back not hurting anymore, Mummy? Can you come to the zoo with us?" my heart tightens. It feels impossible to respond, "Of course, pumpkin!" because the truth is, I cannot.

To shield myself from reigniting my psychological and physical suffering, I avoid anything that might trigger distress: certain photos, places, music, movies, people—even smells. These triggers plunge me into overwhelming emotional turmoil, and my reactions are often vivid and uncontrollable. My mind plays the same obsessive refrain, my rumination ever-present.

Walking in the sleet, when your body feels so weak,
And the sadness in your eyes, you no longer can
disguise.

This constant undercurrent pulls me deeper into depression. The past feels relentless, as if it is chasing me down. Memories of both recent and past traumas haunt me despite my will to break free. When Emily asks to watch a movie like *Cars* or *Rapunzel,* I remember my older children making the same requests. Tears flow as I mourn the days when I could accompany them on their journey to adulthood.

My relationship with Camille suffers deeply under the weight of my depression. Walled in by my sadness, I brood over dark thoughts and interpret every event as a dark omen. I am consumed by doubt and guilt. Unable to trust or open up, I can't re-engage in the closeness we once shared. I fear suffering again—and worse, suffering for the rest of my life. Day by day, I close myself off from him more, further isolating myself.

In February 2023, I began expressive writing workshops—not to relive my traumatic events, but to recreate them. Writing bridges the creative right brain and the logical left brain, using language as a gateway to the imagination. This process allows me to create emotional distance from past events, rewriting them in the present with fresh perspectives and a calmer mind. Through writing, I can confront the past and, in doing so, begin to shape a fulfilling future.

This creative process grants me the freedom to express my deepest emotions and most intimate thoughts without shame or fear of judgment. I strive to be honest, especially when exploring emotions that terrify me. At times, these workshops provoke physical reactions: a sudden migraine or an aching back. Often, I cry deeply. I confront my "shameful self," my fears, my repressed desires, and unmet needs. Despite the discomfort, I remind myself that this confrontation is essential for healing. Facing these emotions, which my brain perceives as threats, is the only way to free myself from their grip.

After fifteen minutes of writing, I invite my rational mind into the conversation. With compassion and kindness, I step back to reflect on what I've written. Guided by my unconscious, I analyze and rationalize my emotions, then symbolically release them by tearing up the pages and throwing them away—a definitive break from their hold over me.

If you are considering freeing yourself from trauma through writing, know that in the beginning, the process may evoke sadness, nostalgia, or even setbacks. At first, I felt as though I was going back to square one, and it was stressful. But over time, I realized this is normal —and a good sign. It means the healing process is underway. As the days passed, the workshops became lighter, and I always made sure to end each session on a note of optimism, focusing on my dreams, hopes, and the bright future I'm working toward.

CHAPTER TWENTY

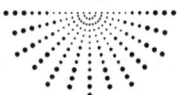

*A*fter freeing myself from my feelings and fears, I now embark on the second daily step of my journey: reprogramming my brain. Pain Reprocessing Therapy (PRT) teaches us that pain is not always a reliable indicator of tissue damage. By breaking this vicious cycle, we reduce the level of perceived danger in the brain, creating a sense of security.

Later in therapy, I began gradually reintroducing movements that caused pain, creating positive corrective experiences. These experiences teach the brain that no movement is inherently dangerous or to be avoided. The body is fine; it's the mind that suffers! Step by step, we reprogram the brain to unlearn fear and take the neural pathways of zero pain once again. Pain, in this sense, is nothing more than the result of a faulty mind-body connection.

When the brain understands that we are aware of what's happening within us and are willing to act, it gradually "turns off" the pain.

As part of my therapy, I volunteered to play the role of the patient during a videoconference for somatic tracking courses. Somatic tracking is a practice that combines mindfulness, reevaluation of perceived dangers, and induction of positive emotions. The idea is to become aware of physical sensations in the body at a given moment, observing them without fear or judgment.

I must admit, it was quite unsettling to sit with my eyes closed, fully aware that more than a hundred people from around the world were watching me—and that the session was being recorded for later replay. Knowing that every move I made was being scrutinized added an unexpected layer of vulnerability to the experience.

John, my trainer, begins by suggesting that I observe my sensations without judgment, in complete safety, and without fear. His approach creates a bridge between pleasant and unpleasant sensations, encouraging me to explore them with curiosity and lightness. As I follow his guidance, I experience a strange shift—it feels as though my brain is gradually becoming less afraid of confronting unpleasant sensations, as if it's learning to coexist with them.

Next, John suggests welcoming my sensations and evaluating them to determine whether they're pleasant or not. With humor and lightness, he reminds me, *"These sensations are just sensations."* He points to the tension in the lower part of my back, explaining that it's simply lumbar tension, the result of a locked muscular chain.

"Lili, have you ever fallen asleep on your arm? What did you feel when you woke up?" he asks.

I recall the numbness and tingling, as if thousands of tiny needles were pricking me.

"You see, Lili, that unpleasant tingling in your back is similar. It's not dangerous. You can accept it for what it is: just a sensation."

At that moment, he encourages me to detach from the unpleasant sensations and focus instead on neutral ones. He also asks me to recount everything that's happened to me recently. As I begin to speak, an unexpected surge of emotions floods through me—anger, shame, guilt, fear, and distress—until I burst into tears, completely overwhelmed and out of words.

"Lili, you must love yourself. You're a kind person, so cultivate that kindness toward yourself. And remember, you have the right to make mistakes!" John's words resonate deeply with me. Just as I learn to accept my sensations, I must also accept my emotions, my traumatic history, and my complicated relationships. He encourages me to observe my automatic behaviors and thoughts without judgment, releasing the pressure I impose on myself. By reducing the overall level of fear in my mind and body, I aim to neutralize chronic pain at its root.

It's a confusing process, but gradually, I notice my back tensions decreasing in intensity—almost disappearing completely. Curiously, I also stop noticing the other students watching me. I am entirely present with my sensations and emotions, as if the world around me has faded away. By the end, I feel completely drained, like I've just crossed the finish line of an 800-meter race. Although the pain later resurfaces, I've touched the cusp of a life without pain.

By shifting my perception, I realize I have the power to transform my experience of pain. When I see how this therapy impacts my pain, it's challenging to limit myself to the recommended one or two sessions per day. The biggest psychological hurdle is not feeling disappointed when the pain inevitably returns. I remind myself to focus on the positive aspects—because somatic tracking *does* work. If I can influence pain in the short term, then, in the long term, I can overcome it.

Thanks to various training sessions, I've regained a social life, even though it remains largely virtual for now. Still, my days are once again filled with experiences I look forward to sharing with Cam. Just like before, we exchange anecdotes at the end of the day, cuddled on the couch once the little one is asleep. Slowly but surely, life is returning to something beautiful and whole.

When I discovered the impact this therapy has on my painful experience, I realized how difficult it is to limit myself to the recommended one or two sessions per day. The biggest psychological challenge is managing the disappointment when the pain inevitably resurfaces. But I remind myself to focus on the positive—because somatic tracking *does* work. If I can influence pain in the short term, I am confident I can overcome it in the long term.

Thanks to various training sessions, I now have a social life again, even if it's still mostly virtual. My days are once more filled with experiences I eagerly look forward to sharing with Cam. Like we used to, we exchange anecdotes at the end of the day, cuddled on the couch after the little one has fallen asleep.

Sharing, discussing, and constructively critiquing ideas stimulate us both. Interestingly, Cam has even heard about brain reprogramming from the coach he collaborates with for his field hockey team's European championships. Together, we are rediscovering precious moments of laughter and intimacy.

I no longer feel like a burden. Instead, I'm starting to feel like myself again—like a woman.

* * *

Today, as I conclude my day—after expressing myself in a writing workshop and reprogramming my brain through PRT—I am preparing to calm my nervous system. Instead of attempting a lengthy meditation session, which I don't feel ready for yet, I focus on cultivating long-term healthy habits. Today, that means embarking on a journey to the land of mindfulness.

The human mind is notoriously difficult to tame. It remembers and projects, regrets and plans, ruminates and anticipates. Meditation, as a holistic practice, is an incredibly effective tool for managing emotions and regulating the mind. It also contributes to neuroplasticity—the brain's ability to rewire itself. According to tradition, it was through this practice that the Buddha is said to have achieved *samādhi*, or enlightenment. Similarly, in the third and fourth centuries, the Desert Fathers encouraged their disciples to meditate, advising them to "sit, be silent, and calm their thoughts."

This ancient practice has proven itself in the modern world, offering a powerful antidote to stress, anxiety, burnout, and chronic pain.

I must admit, I once considered meditation a waste of time. But I've come to understand the importance of cultivating a "correct mind"—a state of clarity and stability essential for making wise decisions in the face of challenges. Meditation isn't about sitting in the Lotus position, breathing strangely, and waiting for divine enlightenment. It's a practical technique for relaxation and mind-training, helping to develop concentration and grounding in the present moment.

The goal is not to control thoughts but to accept them, quelling the mind's restless wandering. My emotions are not my enemies; they are like clouds, drifting above my head, coming and going without permanence.

Meditation also has profound physical benefits. It reduces biological markers of inflammation, aiding the body's recovery after trauma. It stimulates brain functions such as attention, concentration, and memory, while also lowering blood pressure and improving respiratory health.

> *Always running towards a happiness so undefined,*
> *Always waiting in vain for tomorrows somewhere brighter*
> *   to find.*
> *No more seeking solace in this tiny haven of peace,*
> *The utopia of those who own nothing, nothing but their*
> *   dreams.*

In 1979, Jon Kabat-Zinn, a distinguished professor and molecular biologist with a passion for meditation and yoga, observed the profound benefits of mindfulness. He noted significant reductions in stress, anxiety, and mental and physical suffering among his patients. For me, beyond these benefits, meditation serves as a powerful tool to reprogram my brain toward gratitude and compassion.

Consider this: the only difference between saying *"I have to do"* and *"I want to do"* lies in the verb. Yet, this simple shift in perspective can be transformative. The distinction between *"I have to"* and *"I want to"* is often the root of many of our daily struggles. By approaching even the most mundane tasks with enthusiasm, motivation, and joy, we can profoundly influence our emotional state. Fully engaging in these moments creates a ripple effect, turning the ordinary into something extraordinary.

My three-year-old daughter Emily is also on her own journey of learning self-control and managing her emotions—a completely normal process for her age. When she's overcome by a tantrum, I hold her close, place her small hand on my heart so she can feel its rhythm, and gently encourage her to close her eyes and take deep breaths.

This simple practice not only helps her find calm but also transforms her emotional storm into a moment of connection and growth. Through these moments, I see how mindfulness can nurture not just self-awareness but also a deeper bond between us.

Today, a pale ray of sunshine timidly passes through the blinds, and I rise with the firm intention of practicing what I've learned in my mindfulness meditation class. As soon as I wake, I take a deep breath and begin observing my thoughts. An uninterrupted flow of dark thoughts quickly disrupts this precious moment, and tensions insidiously settle in my body.

I gently get up, allowing each muscle the time to stretch. Then, I note down all the thoughts clouding my mind in the notebook on my bedside table. With that release, I take a moment to "STOP," pausing to suspend my five senses and anchor myself in the present moment:

- **Stop.** I close my eyes, grant myself a precious break, and nourish my mind with positivity. I savor this moment, focusing on the rhythm of my breath to calm the incessant flow of thoughts. I welcome these thoughts without judgment, letting them drift away like clouds. Each time my mind strays, I gently bring my attention back to my breath.

- **Take a deep breath.** I inhale and exhale slowly, deliberately. One hand rests on my chest and the other on my belly, which rise and fall with each breath. For about ten breaths, I relish the soothing sensations. The scent of hot coffee wafting from the kitchen adds a pleasant layer to this experience.

- **Observe.** I open my eyes and curiously take in my surroundings as if seeing them for the first time. I focus on small details and select one object to describe out loud—its shape, colors, size, and texture—bringing it to life with my words. I listen, without judgment, to the sounds around me. My attention first lands on the comforting noises from my daughter's room as she gets dressed with her father. Then I hear the cheerful notes of Miley Cyrus' *"Flowers"* playing on the radio. Between the sounds, I focus on the silence that rests in the gaps. I explore textures, noting the sensations where my skin meets the world—the softness of my pajamas, the coolness of the floor beneath my feet. I gently touch and massage my face with my hands, reconnecting with my body and anchoring myself in these physical sensations.

- **Proceed mindfully.** I choose my response to my observations and emotions with intention. My mind will wander—this is normal; it's human. Staying grounded in the present moment takes practice, and while some days it's easier than others, persistence brings progress. With each practice, it becomes more natural to stabilize the mental restlessness and find peace.

I'll admit—it's hard for me to truly do nothing. Even when I claim to, I often catch myself mindlessly scrolling through Instagram or Facebook. That's why I've made a conscious choice to genuinely clear my mind: no thoughts of overdue tasks, no errands, no diving into the digital rabbit hole. One small habit has made a significant difference: when my phone rings, I take a deep breath before looking at it. It's my way of breaking the urgency tied to notifications. Honestly, it's astonishing—maybe even alarming—how much time we lose to these endlessly distracting apps.

Instead of taking my shower with my mind elsewhere, as I used to, I now fully immerse myself in the sensory experience. I observe the warm, soothing water flowing over my skin and let myself be intoxicated by the scent of vanilla and monoï. By gently massaging the painful areas of my body, I reconnect with my physical self, especially my foot, which I had avoided touching since its partial paralysis. *I will love my body again,* I affirm to myself, even if it's not the ideal body I dream of—even if it makes me suffer. When negative thoughts or a vibration from my phone intrude, I bring my attention back to the sound of the flowing water.

During a distance meditation class, my teacher, Rajeev, asked, *"Do you take the time to truly savor a cup of coffee, tea, or water each day?"* We all confidently replied, *"Of course."* But when he clarified that gulping coffee between tasks didn't count, silence fell. I pictured myself: phone in one hand, tea in the other, multitasking like a modern Durga—minus the mindful intention her ten arms might symbolize. I realized I wasn't savoring my tea; I was simply drinking it while mentally racing to the next task.

In my "old" life, I would jump out of bed already juggling my to-do list: grab groceries, update daycare, pack the gym bag… But now, I approach drinking tea with mindfulness, savoring this simple yet profound "cup of life." Comfortably seated with my feet firmly grounded, I take my mug in both hands. Out loud, I describe its color, scent, and temperature, noticing its rich, soothing nuances. I take a sip, close my eyes, and describe the taste, enjoying the aromas that tickle my nostrils. Then I open my eyes and describe my emotions and feelings, rediscovering details I used to overlook.

There are as many ways to meditate as there are meditators. I've learned there's always time for mindfulness meditation—it's *our* top priority of the day. You can practice it anywhere: while brushing your teeth, at work, on public transport, in the car, or even in traffic. When I'm stopped at a red light, instead of letting impatience take over, I focus on my breath and observe my surroundings. *Has this little restaurant always been here?* I've realized I was often running on autopilot. Now, I consciously listen to the radio, trying to distinguish different instruments without letting my mind wander. And when the first notes of *Stairway to Heaven* come on, it's a delightful seven-minute mindfulness challenge I eagerly embrace! Sometimes, I even turn off the music to listen to the sounds of nature behind the city's hum.

When I began meditating, I started with short daily sessions of mindfulness and gradually increased their duration. Barefoot, to feel the connection between my feet and the ground, I sit motionless on a chair or yoga mat. Keeping my back straight and shoulders relaxed, I fix my gaze on a point or half-close my eyes, directing my non-judgmental attention to the present moment. This practice has become an active pause to build resilience, helping me accept my pain for what it is: a misfiring of my brain. My lower back pain is a neural error; the pain in my foot is neuropathic and something I must coexist with.

By ceasing to fight or flee from pain, I've taken a decisive step toward inner harmony, creating the conditions for healing. I now recognize the warning signs of pain and anticipate them, drawing from my zero-pain toolkit. I no longer feel trapped or powerless. My "meditating" brain processes painful emotions without panic, limiting cerebral inflammation.

By mourning the life I once led, I've come to accept that life continues—differently, and sometimes even better.

CHAPTER TWENTY-ONE

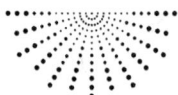

While combating my psychological pain, I also began to tackle my kinesiophobia—an irrational fear of getting injured while moving. The medical community has repeatedly told me that I likely hurt my back by carrying my daughter, and those words have deeply rooted themselves in my memory. Like an insistent refrain, this fear of "dangerous" movement constantly haunts me, giving rise to avoidant behaviors that multiply.

The mere idea of lifting my daughter generates tension in my lower back. These fear-avoidance behaviors stifle my impulses toward enriching activities like hobbies and social interactions. Nevertheless, I am gradually reacquainting my body with all movements, weaving new, positive associations day by day.

Mentioning the resumption of walking abruptly plunges me into memories of my former life—a time when I was immersed in various sports teams and partnerships. I represented Garmin in the Paris Triathlon, Compex in the Paris Marathon, Volkswagen in the Lille Half Marathon, and Saint-Yorre in the Paris 10K. I constantly sought that adrenaline rush, the exhilaration of the starting line, and the thrill of pushing my limits within a team. For as long as I can remember, *sport* has always been synonymous with *performance*. Running was my way of feeling alive, and I loved serving noble causes. One of my most cherished memories is climbing the 1,776 steps of Toronto's CN Tower for WWF.

For a long time, I dismissed walking as a sport. To me, it was simply a way to get from point A to point B or a relaxed Sunday activity with the family. But now, walking is about to become my new sport and personal challenge—and I'm excited.

Then came an unexpected twist: my daughter's daycare temporarily moved to a new building. This change gave me a clear goal—a one-and-a-half-kilometer walk there and back—and a month to prepare. Given my limp, I anticipate the round trip will take about an hour.

Determined to succeed, I've integrated a daily walk into my routine, embracing it as a step toward rebuilding my strength and resilience.

Now, I've incorporated a daily walk into my routine, setting a goal to go a little farther each day. True to my athletic nature, I initially created a training plan with specific objectives: "If I maintain this pace, I'll be walking for an hour in just a few weeks." But some days, I felt strong; others, not at all. This goal-oriented approach quickly led to frustration—and, of course, pain.

The key to transforming these outings from a task into a joy came from what Alan Gordon calls *"outcome independence."* I learned to be satisfied with my actions and efforts, regardless of the final result. In my case, it no longer mattered whether I walked farther or shorter than the day before. My physical goal became secondary, part of a long-term vision rather than a short-term measure of success. The psychological goal, however, became essential.

I now feel happy when I return home, not because I hit a milestone, but because I chatted with a neighbor, soaked up a healthy dose of vitamin D, or listened to a fascinating podcast. Don't get me wrong —I'm not suggesting we abandon goal-setting. On the contrary, goals are vital for growth and self-transcendence. But when we detach ourselves from the outcome and celebrate small steps forward, pain, stress, and pressure gradually loosen their grip.

At this stage, even though I haven't yet conquered the pain completely, its days are undeniably numbered.

* * *

Empowerment—"the taking of power or control"—is a term that deeply resonates with me. To overcome fear and prevent it from resurfacing, one must experience the profound feeling of empowerment. Taking control of one's life, regaining confidence in one's abilities, and realizing the capacity to overcome any obstacle are essential steps. Empowerment brings joy instead of frustration, liberation instead of imprisonment. When I decided that pain would no longer dictate my mood, behavior, or plans, change came quickly.

Regaining control and detaching from the final result allowed me to achieve my goals faster while limiting the impact of disappointments, failures, and loss of motivation along the way. As a result, relapses have much less hold on me.

Athletes know that their opponent is also their greatest partner, as it's the one who drives them to progress. In the same way, I chose to challenge my pain rather than avoid it, facing it with determination. I no longer see pain as an enemy, but as an adversary. And in this contest, may the stronger mind win (spoiler: that's me)! From that moment, my progress accelerated. The more confidently I confronted pain, the less I suffered. My fear of it diminished, replaced by a growing desire to face it head-on and reclaim control of my life.

Every time we succeed at a task, we cultivate what psychologist Albert Bandura calls a *sense of self-efficacy*. The more victories I achieved against pain, the stronger my belief in my ability to overcome it became. Over time, these small wins became the foundation of my growing self-confidence.

Physiologically, celebrating these victories releases dopamine, reinforcing the cycle. Whether I'm facing my fears or finally tackling the paperwork that's been piling up for two weeks, it's a reason to celebrate. What I celebrate isn't just the success itself, but the building block it adds to the structure of my self-confidence. Each win, no matter how small, strengthens my resolve and reminds me that I am in control.

Despite my determination, I feel a wave of anxiety as I set out for my first longer outing in the Citadel woods of Lille, conveniently located at the end of my street. I've worked hard to rebuild the strength in my back, legs, and entire body after months of suffering and bed rest. But as I take my first steps, the initial sensations are far from encouraging.

Pain greets me at every turn—my foot burns, and a lingering, diffuse ache accompanies each step, a constant reminder of my body's new limits. I realize I need to lower my expectations for today. Disappointment creeps in as I turn back, but I am not discouraged.

Some days are better. The pain is less intense, and as it fades, I even feel a glimmer of joy and relief. Yet, the pain always returns, cruelly reminding me of the uphill battle I face. There are days when walking becomes an insurmountable challenge, and I have to turn back just a few meters from home.

Then, troubling new symptoms arise. My left foot alternates between red and blue, icy cold and burning hot. It seems I'm dealing with Raynaud's syndrome, which brings numbness, circulatory issues, and even frostbite on my toes. It feels endless, and for a moment, despair threatens to take hold.

But now, with the emotional strength I've built, I refuse to let pain win. I head to the pharmacy, where my "good fairy" Charlotte suggests an insulating cream. Armed with her advice and my unyielding resolve, I set out again, ready to face adversity. Even if I fall, I get up—literally and figuratively.

Thanks to my ability to detach from the final result, I celebrate each small victory and draw motivation from them. I adjust my goals and set realistic milestones. My sweetheart fully embraces his role as my coach, sometimes accompanying me on my outings. His unwavering belief in me bolsters my determination.

He is certain I will overcome this ordeal—and so am I.

Your confidence in me is such a sight to see,
And you are and will always be the better part of me.
The emptiness I fell when you're not by my side,
The rock that's given me the strength with nothing to hide.

During this same period, I searched tirelessly for a rehabilitation center that could accommodate me, only to face rejection after rejection. After months of persistence, I was finally called for a pre-visit and evaluation at the Les Hautois rehabilitation center in Oignies.

During the interview, the doctor was incredibly encouraging: *"Of course, you will run again! Of course, you'll surf and play tennis!"* His confidence reignited something within me. I seized the opportunity to share my book and the method I had developed. To my delight, he wholeheartedly agreed with my perspective, acknowledging that the future of chronic pain care lies, in part, in harmonizing the body and mind. His words still resonate with me.

Following that consultation, progress came at lightning speed. Was it the doctor's optimism, the placebo effect, or perhaps the looming pressure of the "daycare deadline"? I can't provide a rational explanation, but one thing is certain: those few minutes of walking quickly turned into dozens.

Cam was convinced I could do it, and our shared enthusiasm became contagious. Every additional step became a challenge conquered, a powerful symbol of my rediscovered resilience, and proof that I was once again the master of my fate.

I felt this rebirth most profoundly on the day I saw disbelief, then joy, in my daughter's eyes as she exclaimed, *"Mummy, are you taking me to daycare today?"* Her reaction was my true victory, shining brightly in her gaze—a moment I will carry with me forever.

I now indulge in walking several times a day, regardless of the duration. This simple activity helps me channel my surplus energy. To soothe my nervous system and better manage persistent painful sensations, I sometimes combine my walks with breathing and mindfulness exercises, sitting on a bench under a tree.

Other times, I walk without headphones, focusing instead on my breathing and my steps. I place one foot consciously in front of the other, aware of the momentary imbalance between lifting my foot and placing it back on the ground. Am I afraid of this imbalance? No. I simply observe my still hesitant, limping gait and accept it. I notice the swing of my arms and walk slowly, fully concentrating on my sensations.

Am I cold? Does a breeze brush my face? I resist the urge to think about the grocery list or the laundry. When my mind begins to wander, I welcome the thoughts like clouds drifting across the sky, letting them pass as I refocus on my breath.

I seize every opportunity to walk, whether it's to run errands, visit the post office, or take my daughter to daycare. The warmth of reconnecting with the world is indescribable—like being greeted by the baker exclaiming, *"Oh my God, we haven't seen you in so long!"*

To keep myself motivated, I set small goals and use an app called WeWard, which even converts my daily steps into euros. Slowly but surely, life is resuming its course. We've renewed our subscription to the zoo at the Citadel of Lille for our Sunday walks.

"Mummy, are you coming with us to the zoo?" Emily asks.

For the first time in what feels like forever, I can answer with a confident, *"Of course, little love!"*

CHAPTER TWENTY-TWO

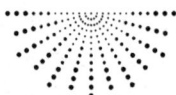

*A*pril, with its sunny days and warmer breezes, brings comfort to my heart. Adding to the joy, Cam decides to sell his house and move in permanently with Emily and me. As the days pass, my routine grows richer with new tools. I express my emotions through art, explore the emotional freedom technique, and work to reprogram my brain to avoid overreacting to everyday stressors. I also strive to follow the principles of neuro-linguistic programming.

The concept of "art therapy" wasn't coined until 1942, when Adrian Hill, a British artist recovering from tuberculosis in a sanatorium, observed—and his caregivers confirmed—that painting and drawing significantly aided his recovery. By the 1950s, formal training programs for art therapists had emerged in the United States, though France didn't officially recognize art therapy as a scientific discipline until the 1980s. Two main approaches developed: traditional art therapy, practiced by psychotherapists, and "modern" art therapy, a distinct paramedical discipline. It was the latter path I chose when I enrolled in the university diploma program at the Free Faculty of Medicine in Lille.

However, when I began proposing art therapy workshops to

various institutions, I quickly encountered resistance and misconceptions:

"Hello, my name is Lili Road, and I am an art therapist. I'd like to propose art therapy sessions for your institution."

"Oh, that's for children—our elderly audience won't like it."

"Actually, art therapy today is applied in a variety of settings: geriatric services, prisons, and even among homeless populations."

"Oh, thanks, but we already have art classes."

"Art therapy isn't the same as art classes. In art therapy workshops, the goal isn't to improve artistic techniques but to use the therapeutic properties of art to support emotional and psychological well-being."

"Well, since it's not a proven therapy, we'd prefer to allocate funds elsewhere. Thanks again."

* * *

When we were young students, what were our favorite moments in school? Drawing, coloring, painting, singing, and dancing. These were the activities that made us happy, filled us with pride, and left us eager to share our creations with our parents. Yet, as the years passed, these joyful moments gradually disappeared from our lives.

So, isn't it time to bring back that spark of creativity and playful lightness into our daily routines?

Reviving true colors, soft and bright shadows,
Life springs forth in verdant grass,
From a white canvas, from a black canvas,
From a canvas of black and white,
Shaping works of art.

What excites me most about art therapy is the belief that we are all artists. As an art therapist, my primary role is to establish a trusting relationship with my patients, reassuring them that they don't need to be "good" at art to benefit from its therapeutic virtues. "Can't draw? That's not a problem—neither can I!" We all have an artistic soul and potential that can serve as a powerful tool for healing.

The uniqueness of art therapy lies in its use of art as an integral part of the healing process, employing various techniques such as drawing, painting, music, dance, singing, calligraphy, or writing. Each art therapy session is therefore as unique as the individual it supports.

Practicing art therapy means letting go—allowing the pencil to move across the paper without engaging the analytical brain or inviting judgment. It's about experiencing art as a living expression, rooted in the body and soul. Art therapy helps to bring forth what lies dormant within us, including the darkest emotions. Through art, we unlock the doors to our authentic selves.

Words often fail to express the full scope of repressed traumas. Psychological pain is sometimes stored in our memory as sensations and emotions, not as narratives. When we attempt to articulate these sufferings verbally, we often reach an impasse, confronting the unspeakable. Georgia O'Keeffe captured this beautifully: *"I noticed that I could say things with colors and shapes for which I had no words."*

Through the art therapy sessions I've facilitated, I've learned to adorn unpleasant sensations with colors, taming and transforming them. I've sublimated my pain into unique, symbolic creations, giving hue and shape to the intangible feelings that once haunted me. Drawing the monsters from "under the bed" shouldn't be reserved for children; it's an act of exorcising inner demons that is profoundly healing.

For those living with chronic pain, consciousness often oscillates between moments of happiness and the shadow of pain, until the pain eventually consumes everything, tinting life black. What emotions do certain colors evoke in me? Colors have a language of their own. From advertisers to architects, countless professions harness the symbolism of colors to influence our emotions. Art therapy allows us to reclaim this power, using color and form to process and heal.

Finding pleasure in creating a vibrant artistic mosaic as an acknowledgment of my pain counters the tyranny it imposes. Art therapy workshops are far from somber moments. Yes, there have been tears, but they've been accompanied by bursts of laughter and moments of joy.

By trusting my intuition during the creative process, I also nourish my self-confidence. I've even experimented with drawing and painting in the dark or with my eyes covered. The surprise is always remarkable when we uncover what our emotions have been waiting to reveal to us.

* * *

Pain is not me, and I am not my pain. Art provides a way to distance ourselves from internal conflicts, creating a neutral space to explore emotional blockages. It serves as both a medium for expressing the authentic self and a creative outlet. The heart—sometimes heavy, sometimes light, and often a bit of both—holds everything that animates us. In the Latin sense of the term, it encompasses everything that breathes soul into our existence.

But what exactly resides within the heart? Our children? Our spouse? Sports? Our four-legged companions? Outings with friends? Chronic pain? Excessive stress at work? Using drawings, colors, words, and collages to create varied textures, I enjoy mapping out what is most important to me. Revisiting these creations at regular intervals helps me better understand myself, track the evolution of my priorities, and observe the space pain occupies in my life.

This process feels deeply familial, and I especially value sharing it with my little one. In institutions, I've also used this tool with adolescents, whose heightened sensitivity often makes understanding and managing emotions a complex challenge.

While searching for inspiration for new workshops, I came across a study whose findings immediately resonated with me. At a pain management center in New Zealand, participants were invited to visually represent their pain and then write the story behind their creation. Each experience took shape through colors, forms, and words, revealing themes that I, too, have encountered: the loss of self, the redefinition of identity, and the relentless struggle to maintain hope.

Surprisingly, some participants also unearthed positive aspects, reframing the experience of chronic pain as an odyssey—a journey of resilience, discovery, and transformation.

And indeed, that's how I came to view this (mis)adventure—as an initiatory journey. Forced to slow down, I took the time to reflect on what truly matters. The troubles of the body mirrored the troubles of the soul, teaching me that living fully is about savoring each moment. It is the act of *"being"* rather than *"doing"* that opens the door to happiness.

Interestingly, this realization was not entirely new to me. Back in 2013, I had already expressed it in the lyrics of my song, *"When the Storm Breaks"*:

Renew the authenticity of instants drifting in decay,
A sea of surplus on the way, where true essence fades away.

Only ten years later do I truly grasp its meaning. During this journey, I realized that my greatest enemy was fear—fear of pain, fear of movement, and, most of all, fear of fully experiencing my emotions. Reintroducing writing and art into my daily life became transformative, allowing me to create a cocoon of physical and psychological safety for my brain.

Words on the pains, colors for the strain,
Music for healing, a comforting refrain.

Art—whether expressed through colors or notes—acts as a decompression chamber, an open door to another world. Gradually, through writing, art, and music, my brain begins to relax, releasing the pressure tied to the psychological dangers it perceives.

* * *

One day in late April, I received an invitation from Yoga Alliance, where I'm a member and a yoga and meditation teacher, to attend a conference on the Emotional Freedom Technique (EFT). Intrigued by its potential—particularly in the context of chronic pain—I eagerly seized the opportunity to learn more.

EFT, founded in 1995, emerged from the intersection of classical psychotherapy, particularly the theory of conditioned responses, and traditional Chinese medicine's meridian system used in acupuncture.

Developed by Gary Craig, EFT builds on Roger Callahan's earlier work in phobia healing. Craig simplified the original techniques, integrating them with behavioral and cognitive therapies. As a result, EFT combines trauma exposure, cognitive restructuring, and somatic stimulation of acupressure points on the face and body.

The goal of EFT is to restore balance between the body and mind by addressing energy disturbances caused by negative thoughts, painful events, or physical and psychological traumas. Initially, I found the concept somewhat abstract, but in practice, it's a very concrete therapy. Negative emotions such as fear, anger, and guilt are believed to create blockages in the body's energy pathways. By tapping on specific acupressure points, EFT helps release these blockages and restore the body's energy flow.

I understand that terms like "meridians" and "energy flow" might raise skepticism. However, in countries where pharmaceutical sales are significantly lower than ours, such concepts are an integral part of medical terminology and practice.

Although I approached EFT with some initial reservations, I quickly recognized its potential. Over a hundred studies have demonstrated its effectiveness in addressing both physiological and psychological symptoms. It proved to be an excellent complement to the emotional empowerment workshops I had already been implementing.

Encouraged by the insights from the conference, I decided to dive deeper into EFT the following week. After all, I had nothing to lose— it's a technique with no associated risks, and the potential benefits were too significant to ignore.

He was so different from before,
because his mind never returned from the war.
It was as if my love had died, and yet there was no grave.

Eager to deepen my knowledge, I enrolled in a masterclass with Dr. Gupta. True to form, I seized the opportunity to test this therapeutic tool live, and I was amazed by my experience during the session. We focused on my fear of movement and explored the possibility that I might be punishing myself indirectly. Could my suffering and deprivation of pleasure be a way to alleviate the guilt I still feel for not having been more resilient to stress? By continuing to suffer, was I subconsciously justifying my inability to be everywhere and handle everything?

Beyond the odd sensation of tapping the top of my head while repeating Dr. Gupta's words, I experienced a full spectrum of emotions —from laughter to tears—and even, for a moment, forgot the pain. Most importantly, I felt a breakthrough: I was ready to resume more intense physical activities. Was it a placebo effect? Perhaps. A coincidence? I can't say. What I do know is that in the same week, buoyed by my test results, my physiotherapist suggested a more rigorous training regimen, including squats, push-ups, and planks.

What fascinates me about the Emotional Freedom Technique is its emphasis on the connection between body and mind as the center-piece of healing. I use the power of my mind through self-suggestion while simultaneously tapping on my body. This simple, easy-to-learn technique came at just the right time. My brain still associates physical movement with pain, and it's now my job to prove that assumption wrong.

From now on, I turn to "rounds" of tapping whenever pain inten-sity increases. The signals sent to my brain through my fingers and words work to break the association between "emotion and danger" and "pain and danger," replacing them with a new association: "emo-tion, pain, safety." Whenever old, negative patterns reappear, I rely on daily tapping rounds to counteract them. I've embraced my role as an active participant in my healing process.

My personality has been shaped by many factors. While some traits are innate, much of who I am has been molded by my upbringing and the socio-economic environment of my childhood. Similarly, pain has become so deeply rooted in me that it feels almost intrinsic to my identity. It has given rise to a pessimism that inclines me to see the glass as half empty, perpetuating the cycle of chronic pain.

The traumas I've endured have also fostered personality traits like lack of self-confidence, hypersensitivity, hyperemotionality, and alter-nating phases of hyperactivity and depression. I won't attempt to erase these traits—they are integral to who I am and, as my darling says, part of my charm. However, I will observe them closely, along with the automatic thoughts they generate, so I can retain their benefits without being burdened by their drawbacks.

As a perfectionist, I often viewed pain management in extremes: either rest and leave tasks unfinished, or push forward at a frantic pace with the help of painkillers. Growing up with a mother who suffered from debilitating migraines, I likely felt an early sense of responsibility as an only child to avoid adding stress to our home. This pressure to be "perfect" led me to become fiercely independent and self-reliant from a young age.

As an adult, this tendency often backfires. I take on too much, bury myself under a mountain of tasks, and leave little time for self-care. The result? I'm constantly on the brink of imploding or exploding. I spend so much time trying to satisfy others that I rarely meet my own needs. Living in a state of chronic stress, I frequently set goals that exceed my resources, unwittingly conditioning my body to create and amplify pain.

Perfectionism is a recurring trap for me. My brain rarely pauses, and when I began developing my method, writing consumed my thoughts day and night. My mind was constantly churning, leading to restless nights filled with doubts, backaches, and the occasional burst of enthusiasm with ideas for the next day's pages.

Through Emotional Empowerment (EE) workshops, I explored this personality trait and discovered that I could ease my perfectionism without compromising my conscientiousness. I still take pride in being efficient and skilled, but I've learned that perfectionism itself isn't inherently a flaw—it's all about finding balance.

To regain control, I decided to stop overinvesting in less important activities and prioritize myself. I planned structured writing sessions and incorporated moments of decompression into my schedule, such as meditation, physiotherapy, and playing the piano. These well-being moments are now non-negotiable.

I've also stopped worrying about trivial things, like how my living room looks when my physiotherapist arrives. Letting go of these small stressors has been liberating and essential to my healing process.

* * *

I've always tended to seek approval from those around me—a survival strategy I developed to avoid conflict. While this approach helped me navigate challenging times, I've come to realize it's unsustainable in the long run. It creates enormous social pressure, leaving me feeling overwhelmed, exploited, and disrespected.

Perhaps you're like me—someone who endures at the expense of their physical and mental health. You might be the one who always says yes, lends a hand in tough times, and helps others with a smile. When my pain intensified, I felt an overwhelming guilt about being less efficient in my family and professional life, as if my reduced productivity was a betrayal of those around me.

During our EFT session, Dr. Gupta picked up on this pattern. Despite suffering, I was driven by a fear of rejection or disappointment to say yes to every thankless task. This tendency to overcommit meant that when I could no longer help everyone or accomplish meaningful tasks, the impact was devastating. I became trapped in a cycle of feeling I needed to constantly prove my worth.

I'm fortunate to have a darling who cooks excellent meals. Yet, my automatic responses to even the simplest questions illustrate my struggle with assertiveness:

"Lili, should I make a flan or a chocolate mousse for dessert?"

"Whatever you want!"

Or,

"Honey, are you hungry?"

"So-so!" (Camille finds this answer particularly amusing.)

By responding this way, I lose sight of my own desires to the point where I can no longer discern what's truly beneficial for me. This lack of clarity reflects a deeper issue: the failure to prioritize my own needs.

It's a truth I've come to understand: I am the most important person in my life, just as you are the most important person in yours. To truly care for others, we must first prioritize our own needs and values. I should have paid more attention to the advice flight attendants give before every flight: *In the event of cabin depressurization, put on your own oxygen mask before assisting others.*

"I really need to nail this presentation in front of my colleagues."

"I should lose some weight before summer."

"I have to clean up before my in-laws arrive this weekend."

These thoughts might seem harmless on paper, but they have a bomb-like effect on the brain. When we hear a negative thought or self-criticism, our brain reacts as though it's under physical attack.

In truth, no personality trait is inherently good or bad. Understanding ourselves means recognizing the mechanisms behind our automatic thoughts, allowing us to anticipate them and avoid their negative consequences. My perfectionism and perseverance, for instance, helped me recover from the bitter failure of my oral exams for the teaching qualification in my first year. But it was through moderation and constructive self-criticism that I succeeded the following year.

CHAPTER TWENTY-THREE

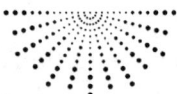

"*C*an you pick up the kids tonight? I can't make it—I finish at 7:30 p.m."

"The grades must be entered into the system by the end of the week. I know the deadlines are tight, but the parent–teacher conferences are coming up."

"Mom, it's Charlotte's birthday tomorrow, remember? Did you buy the pink Magic Unicorn we saw in that store? Ugh, I can't remember which one!"

What happens within us when we hear these everyday demands? What do we feel? A twinge of stress? A gust of panic? A rush of adrenaline or the faint stirrings of a headache? Stress is an inherent part of modern Western life—a normal and, at times, useful reaction to environmental stimuli.

Dr. Hans Selye, a renowned endocrinologist, described stress as a motivational factor, stating: *"Stress is the body's reaction to changes, demands, constraints, or threats in the environment, with the aim of adapting to them."* In other words, stress is the reason you and I are here today. Our ancestors relied on it to escape predators and survive.

However, in our daily lives, stress is often triggered by less life-threatening yet equally demanding scenarios—unforeseen events, tight deadlines, or major life changes like renovating a house, starting a new job, or welcoming a new baby. For modern humans, almost anything can become a source of stress.

While stress can be beneficial in small doses, pushing us to adapt and meet challenges, it can also disrupt the body's balance and become harmful when it exceeds a certain threshold. Understanding this fine line is key to managing stress effectively and ensuring it remains a motivator rather than a burden.

The advent of new technologies has drastically increased the amount of information we consume daily. In fact, we likely process more information in a single day than our grandparents did over the course of their entire lives.

All is quick, all is known—what's left to hold on to?
Life's a rush, always on the go—does anyone truly care
for you?
Clicks and likes, friends and fans, drowned in the
endless "me too."

One thing is certain: I'm well-acquainted with good stress—the kind I feel just before going on stage. It starts with my mind envisioning the worst: forgetting my lyrics or chords, losing my composure. My thoughts race uncontrollably, making it difficult to stay calm. Gradually, this stress manifests physically: my heart pounds, my breathing quickens, my muscles tense. My hands grow sweaty, butterflies flutter in my stomach, and during particularly important concerts, I've even felt nauseous.

Yet, I need this adrenaline rush—this surge of stage fright before the curtain rises—to summon the courage required to perform. It's what keeps me from fleeing in those final minutes before a concert. This mechanism, perfectly tuned to threats or challenges requiring an immediate action–reaction response, is essential for my performance.

This good stress, known as *eustress*, may cause temporary psychosomatic symptoms, but it also allows us to tap into our full physical and intellectual potential to meet a challenge. Once the moment passes, the stress subsides, enabling us to regain physical and mental balance until the next surge comes. When managed effectively, stress can be a powerful ally.

While good stress motivates us, bad stress drains us. In our daily lives, we rarely face mortal dangers. Instead, our stresses are largely psychological: a demanding boss, traffic jams, or the rising cost of living. This is when stress becomes harmful. It lingers, evolving into an unrelenting daily pressure, making recovery difficult, if not impossible.

For me, having removed my two main outlets—sports and music —I turned to my third refuge: food, which had long been a source of emotional comfort. I found myself trapped in a cycle of eating without hunger to fill an emotional void, followed by periods of restriction in an attempt to regain control over my life. Overwhelmed by the mounting responsibilities I faced and the constant tension within my family, I struggled to adapt. This ultimately led to a state of complete exhaustion.

Cam and I lived for years in a state of chronic stress that wore us down emotionally and physically. It tested our resilience, patience, and relationship to its limits. To preserve our children's emotional well-being, we decided not to uproot them, choosing instead to maintain two separate households. However, this decision came at a steep cost. When sick leave began to disrupt our finances, we faced the burden of exorbitant medical expenses while coping with a significantly reduced income.

Our life's structure made day-to-day management complex and time-consuming. Even leisure activities or family outings required meticulous planning to accommodate everyone's needs, making it nearly impossible to please everyone. We exhausted ourselves. Though our relationship weathered the storm, it came at a significant cost. This life was far from the one we had envisioned.

A major contributor to chronic stress is what Frederic Luskin calls "unenforceable rules." According to Luskin, we are the true architects of our stress, exhausting ourselves by clinging to frustrations over situations we cannot control. For example, I wish my house could remain as tidy as it was before we had children. While this is a reasonable desire, my mind often twists it into a demand, turning "I would like …" into "I need …."

Learning to accept certain realities is essential. Even Marie Kondo, the famed queen of Japanese tidying, has admitted that she let go of her ideal of a perfectly organized home after the birth of her third child. If even Marie Kondo allows herself this grace, surely, I can too.

CHAPTER TWENTY-FOUR

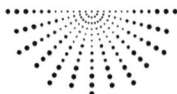

*D*uring my research, I discovered that neuro-linguistic programming (NLP) enabled 76% of individuals to overcome their claustrophobia and calmly undergo an MRI—an exam that was once impossible for them (Bigley et al., 2010). This approach helps individuals regain control of anxiety-inducing situations and fosters a greater sense of mastery over their own lives. Perfect, considering that anxiety and fear are my two sworn enemies. So, in March 2023, still significantly limited in my activities, I seized the opportunity to take a distance learning course in NLP.

NLP originated in the United States in the 1970s. It combines the nervous system (neuro) and the art of language (linguistic) to reshape our internal sensory representations (program), enabling us to achieve our goals more effectively. Gustafson and Lipton (2017) observed: "The brain is equivalent to a computer: it needs a startup system and programs to function. During the first seven years of life, it downloads behaviors by observing what is happening around it. [...] After the age of 7, we start using these programs, but [...] unfortunately, if the programs we received are 'bad,' the conscious mind will self-sabotage without understanding why."

Our worldview is unique, and language—both verbal and nonverbal—reflects this reality by creating distinctive images in our minds. For example, if I say "flower," what comes to mind? I imagine a rose, but you might visualize a tulip. My map (representation) of the territory (reality) is unique and does not align with an objective reality. In essence, there is only one territory but a multitude of maps. Consequently, our actions and reactions are shaped by our individual realities, which explains why it is often challenging to understand someone else's choices, even when they are made sincerely.

NLP offers a fascinating promise: to reprogram our brain by modifying our internal map and choosing a more effective one. If a behavior doesn't help us achieve our goals, NLP suggests that instead of lowering our ambitions, we can change the behavior itself. According to this perspective, failure doesn't exist; there are only opportunities for personal development.

A concrete example of the impact of language can be seen in the pain-related lexicon I use throughout the day. Over time, these words create negative programs in my brain and reinforce neural pathways associated with fear and pain. To counteract this, mentioning the word "pain" or any related qualifiers is now forbidden in my home. This doesn't mean denying pain's existence but rather not allowing it to dominate. A striking example of language's influence on pain perception comes from a study by Koyama et al. (2005). Researchers applied strong, medium, or low heat to volunteers' legs. During the first application, they accurately announced the heat level. During the second, they claimed the heat would be low, even though it was actually more intense. Remarkably, perceived pain decreased by 28% when the heat was described as low.

"I think, I believe, and therefore I am." Since completely avoiding mention of my pain is nearly impossible, I've adopted a lighthearted emergency word: "pelican." This allows me to reference pain without triggering an alarm state in my brain. This approach benefits not only me but also those around me, as talking about chronic pain daily can create an anxious atmosphere at home. Importantly, I also consider the impact of these words on my little one—words of fear and pain can leave a lasting impression.

At first, using "pelican" felt a bit artificial, but it's been effective.

The word has brought some much-needed laughter, and ultimately, isn't that the goal? To bring joy to my brain and divert it from pain. When I use frightening words, I validate painful feelings and unsettle my mind. In contrast, by replacing them with a word that elicits a smile, I reassure my brain and reduce the perceived pain.

* * *

Do you know what an "emotional parasite" is? Thanks to NLP, I discovered that we are all unknowingly infected by one. These emotional parasites manifest as repetitive, inappropriate behaviors we unconsciously adopt—often for years—to mask the emotions we truly feel in the present moment. The term "parasite" also refers to background noise that disrupts communication, and similarly, these emotional parasites create interference, making our emotions harder for others to read. This often leads to emotional misunderstandings, further reinforcing the feeling of being misunderstood—a sentiment already strong for those who feel stigmatized by their painful experiences.

In my NLP workshops, I explored several types of emotional parasites. Among them are:

- The "elastic": An emotion distorted by trauma that resurfaces with the same intensity whenever reactivated.
- The "racket": A substitute emotion that hides the true underlying feeling.
- The "stamp": An explosive emotion triggered by a minor incident, stemming from accumulated frustrations or unexpressed feelings.

Of all these, the "stamp" resonated with me most deeply. When frustration or unspoken emotions pile up, we metaphorically add another "stamp" to our collection, day after day. Some people "explode" regularly, releasing their accumulated emotions, while others bury them until their body, through chronic pain, reminds them that their collection has reached its limit.

Take this scenario:

"Can you drive the kids again on Saturday? I'm going to sports!"

"Okay!" (But in reality, it wasn't okay. I had planned to go shopping instead.)

I fall squarely into the category of "people pleasers"—those who constantly strive to satisfy everyone around them. This behavior has contributed significantly to my stamp collection, and it's a long one. That's why a single additional stamp, one more drop of water, can cause the glass to overflow.

The crown jewel of my impressive collection? Chronic pain. It's my body's way of rewarding years of suppressing negative emotions and ignoring my own needs.

I realized it was essential to learn to set boundaries to manage my daily stress and emotions. Saying yes when I want to say no breeds frustration, resentment, and pain. Moreover, the more we do, the more is expected of us. Some people resort to the "broken plate" technique: deliberately breaking a plate when asked to do the dishes so they won't be asked again. While effective, this doesn't align with my values. Instead, I aim to set natural, respectful limits, say no when necessary, and earn respect without resorting to manipulation.

Nonviolent communication (NVC) has provided me with valuable tools to remove the final barriers that hinder the free and immediate expression of my emotions. NVC replaces the language of blame and judgment with one of kindness and compassion. This shift eliminates the need to suppress spontaneous emotions or mask them with parasitic ones, allowing for more authentic and effective communication.

For example, saying, "I see that your room is messy. I would like to vacuum. Can you put all your stuffed animals in the basket and the toys in the chest under your bed? Thank you, Bunny!" is much more effective than "Bunny, tidy your room, please; I need to vacuum." Similarly, instead of saying, "I would like to do half an hour of yoga. Can you take care of the children, please?"—which opens the door to a potential "Later" or "No"—I can say, "I would like to do half an hour of yoga, please. When are you available to take care of the children?" This phrasing encourages a positive and collaborative response.

When working under pressure, establishing an internal dialogue becomes crucial to release tension. I've often found myself in "nervous peril" situations, rushing to complete a project, only to realize later that no one had respected the deadlines and the project had been postponed. This doesn't mean adopting a careless attitude or neglecting deadlines but rather allowing myself to be human.

This process of introspection may seem overly simplistic on paper, but in practice, our brain engages in similar processes unconsciously. Since my brain sometimes errs in its judgments, I see it as my duty to help it rationalize situations. After expressing my emotions through art and reprogramming my brain through NLP, I am now focused on calming my mind in the long term by reducing the pressures I impose on myself.

In the past, I had already recognized the importance of changing certain habits to feel more fulfilled and effective. Unfortunately, the Covid-19 years, coupled with family troubles, derailed my resolutions. Letting go of dreams or putting them on hold is never easy. When I gave up on music, it wasn't a decision I made lightly; it was a consequence of life's challenges and the inherent uncertainty of an artist's profession. Though it wasn't a joyous choice, I decided to pivot and resume my studies to prepare for the English CAPES (a competitive exam for secondary school teaching).

As a child, I had only one dream: to become a singer. Yet, when asked what I wanted to do in life, I would always say, "an English teacher." I suppose this response reassured my parents—and perhaps myself too. After all, teaching is a more conventional and less precarious career path. My mother's influence as a teacher likely also played a role in sparking my desire to teach. I had been well-prepared for the role; not one of her lesson plans went unused, as I carefully archived them for my stuffed animal "classes."

Now, I am determined to take control of my future: I will become an English teacher. Unfortunately, as often happens, administrative hurdles stand in the way. Convinced that the teacher shortage would make my case compelling, I went directly to the Employment Center to meet with an advisor, hoping my training request to prepare for the CAPES would be welcomed with open arms.

* * *

"I would like to register to prepare for the CAPES and become an English teacher."

"Oh, well, no, Madame, training to prepare for the CAPES is not covered. However, you can prepare for the agrégation if you wish."

I was dumbfounded. The response seemed entirely illogical, especially when comparing the success rates of the CAPES and the agrégation! I had assumed the Employment Center's goal was to ensure the employability of its registrants. Nevertheless, in September, I found myself sitting among perfectly bilingual students in the lecture halls of the University of Lille, ready to take on this unexpected challenge.

Months passed, and I hung on. I had lived in Canada; surely, I could manage this! But midway through the first semester, I was summoned and told I didn't meet the required level for the courses. It was a heavy blow, especially as I was already painfully aware of my shortcomings. There's a significant difference between "knowing how to speak English" and having an in-depth knowledge of Henry James or the Thatcher years.

To clarify: I wasn't preparing for the agrégation but the CAPES. However, the Employment Center required me to attend agrégation-level courses. As they say, "Those who can do more can do less."

Looking back, I am surprisingly grateful for the Employment Center's inconsistencies. This year turned out to be truly remarkable. I've rarely learned so much in such a short period. My unconventional ideas even brought a bit of levity to the polite, serious world of literature students.

For instance, when analyzing a poem that mentioned a chameleon, I couldn't resist referencing Boy George's song. Of course, that chameleon wasn't exactly the one expected in the analysis of a future English agrégée's poem. Or maybe it was...

At the time, the absence of music in my life was undeniably painful, but I didn't have the luxury of feeling sorry for myself. Instead, I threw myself into my studies, working day and night, striving to ingest quotes and dates by the mile—sometimes to the point of mental indigestion. Over time, bonds were formed with professors who saw me struggling, fighting not to sink.

Then came the written exams for admission to the agrégation. Against all odds, I passed! Who could have believed it? I was going to Paris to take the oral tests. I presented myself as I was, but it didn't take long to realize I didn't fit the established codes. Dare I even mention my grades? (Let's just say my highest score was a 5, but shh, let's keep that between us—I must maintain my reputation with my future students.) It was a humbling and stinging setback.

On the bright side, preparing for the agrégation while also taking the CAPES turned out to be a blessing in disguise. The CAPES felt like a breeze by comparison, and I secured first place in France! Now, I'm back at the very high school where I was once a student—not all memories from those days are fond ones, forcing me to confront my demons and exorcise them. Still, being on the other side of the fence has its perks, including reuniting with teachers I deeply appreciated back then.

Balancing three lives in one, however, is no small feat. Half my week is dedicated to my primary teaching load, working with students across four different specialties—a demanding task for someone new to high school teaching. The other half of the week is spent at the teacher training school, where I'm juggling an immense workload, including the preparation of a reflective essay.

And because I apparently enjoy challenges, I've also enrolled as a distance student at the University of Nanterre to take another shot at the agrégation. What a strange idea! My disastrous results in the oral exam should have served as a reality check, but no—I persist. This time, I'm determined to approach the test with a completely different strategy.

On top of all this, I have two children at home, and my days are still only twenty-four hours long. Clearly, I'll need to organize myself better—or, at the very least, differently!

The previous year, I worked around the clock—twenty-four hours a day, seven days a week—surviving on protein bars while poring over my notes in the university library. Yet, despite my relentless effort, I never managed to complete all my planned tasks. This constant shortfall left me stressed and frustrated. If you can relate, welcome to the stressed club!

Modern life demands proactivity and optimal time management, so I embraced multitasking—a concept marketed in management class as a key to happiness and success. However, that myth quickly crumbled, and burnout loomed large. I came to the bitter realization that I wasn't really multitasking. My brain was simply switching rapidly between tasks, which was both exhausting and highly inefficient. I'd drive my little one to school while sending an email, all the while mentally planning dinner. The result? Oops—I still had the cafeteria check in my pocket, forgot the email attachment, and left the shopping list on the kitchen table.

One strategy that helped me immensely in earning the English agrégation and avoiding a repeat of last year's burnout was the Pomodoro Technique. If, like me, you're not Italian and have no clue what "pomodoro" means, it translates to "tomato." In the late 1980s, a student named Francesco Cirillo developed this time-management method, inspired by kitchen timers shaped like tomatoes, to organize study sessions.

When I began applying this technique to my revisions, I was amazed! I became more focused, efficient, and productive. Most importantly, I no longer ended my days with that overwhelming sense of frustration. Its effectiveness has even been confirmed by neuroscientists, and it can be applied both professionally and personally. After all, accumulated stress and the guilt of poorly completed tasks can contribute to chronic pain.

Now, I've shifted my approach: I learn less, but I learn deeper. First, I plan my tasks and prioritize them by importance. Then, I work in focused twenty-five-minute intervals, avoiding distractions and letting my mind wander only during scheduled five-minute breaks. I steer clear of social media during breaks to avoid stretching them longer than intended. Why twenty-five minutes? That's the average time the brain can maintain optimal focus.

To manage interruptions, I keep Post-its handy—when something comes to mind, I jot it down without dwelling on it. After four work cycles, I take a longer, twenty-five-minute break. These breaks are not wasted time; they prevent mental exhaustion. Like a machine, the brain can overheat if pushed too long without rest. So during breaks, I move, relax, and entertain myself!

I've also made it a habit to eliminate distractions, particularly my phone—that ultimate attention magnet. On average, we gain 26% productivity when our phone isn't within reach. Plus, it takes an average of twenty-three minutes and fifteen seconds to refocus after an interruption (Kaspersky Lab, 2016).

The Pomodoro Technique has not only improved my productivity but also my mental well-being. I've learned that working smarter—not harder—is the real secret to success.

* * *

While writing this book, I even placed a note on my door that read: "Do not disturb. Thank you," to ward off real estate agents and salesmen. This level of discipline was unthinkable for me the previous year; I would have considered such breaks a waste of time. Yet now, I realize that working this way has made me more productive, and, as a bonus, my migraines no longer plague me.

And now—the results of the written exams are in. Unbelievable! I'm eligible again, which fills me with a small but well-earned sense of pride. Waking up at five in the morning, studying before the children are awake and before heading to work, then resuming revisions at 8:00 p.m. until I fall asleep—sometimes literally—while working on my British civilization coursework at two in the morning... It hasn't been easy.

At this pivotal moment, a stroke of luck comes into play. I eagerly share the good news with my professors at the University of Lille, knowing it's partly thanks to them. Shortly afterward, I receive a message from Mr. Stevens, my favorite literature professor, offering to help me with a "colle," or practice oral exam. While I lack neither the desire nor the commitment, finding time in both of our schedules is no small feat. But a good coach can change the course of a match, and opportunities like this should not be missed.

Mr. Stevens and I meet at a bar called the Three Brewers, near

Lille-Flandres station. We only have two hours because he has a train to catch. I present the analysis I've prepared on a passage from *Crossing the River* by Caryl Phillips. He listens attentively and provides detailed feedback, revealing nuances and insights I hadn't considered. That day, I don't just drink my refreshing beer; I drink in his wisdom, furiously scribbling notes. The excerpt I analyzed begins with "house" and ends with "home," a deliberate choice by the author to explore themes of belonging and family. Together, we dissect this concept thoroughly.

Then comes the much-anticipated main test. The theme for my seven-hour written exam? (Drumroll, please): "Home" in *Crossing the River* by Caryl Phillips. I am speechless. Out of six books in the program and countless possible topics, this is the one. Luck is smiling on me.

With the agrégation secured, I apply to teach English and management in English at the University of Lille. Of course, I hear the familiar refrain: "The English agrégation at your age? With children and a job? You're wasting your time."

But I've proven them wrong. Without migraines, free from unnecessary pressure, and armed with effective work methods and stress management techniques, I've achieved what many deemed impossible.

Now, with a baby on the way, a new job, and life smiling at me, Cam and I are brimming with excitement for our growing family and future plans. Enthusiasm is contagious, and our projects seem boundless. This is the mindset I had in 2019—the mindset I'm rediscovering, step by step, thanks to the MBC method program.

PART IV
THE SUMMER OF MY LIFE GENTLY BEGINS

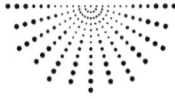

So lay down your suitcase, here and now,
Isn't this the moment to shape our vow?
Cast off the doubts that cloud your perception,
In the core of life, try to find perfection.
So, luv', with a light heart, here and now,
Darlin', by my side, so carefree somehow.

CHAPTER TWENTY-FIVE

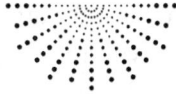

hen I embarked on writing my story, I was convinced that my years on the road as an artist would flow immediately. However, it turned out to be one of the sections I had the most difficulty writing. I faced the complexity of summarizing in a few lines so many memories, encounters, and special moments.

So, I'll start from the beginning. Why suddenly decide to make the stage my profession when I'd never before dared to take the plunge? One day, in October 2010, a few days after my birthday, I received an unexpected gift. A man named Jérôme sent me a message on my Facebook account. He expressed his interest in my songs and proposed a collaboration with Michael Jones, the singer, composer, and guitarist for Jean-Jacques Goldman (an immensely popular singer-songwriter and record producer). It was an extraordinary opportunity for me. Jérôme invited me to a music event at Le Réservoir in Paris, where he promised to introduce me to Michael.

After a long workday, I made my way to Paris. At the end of the show, Michael invited me to join the artists at a nearby restaurant. During the meal, he pulled out his guitar and began improvising on "Hotel California" by the Eagles. Everyone joined in, humming along, and so did I. Before leaving, Michael handed me his email address, asking me to send him my songs because he wanted to listen to them at home. At that moment, I assumed he was just being polite.

But the next day, I received a message from him saying that he was looking forward to hearing my work. Overwhelmed with excitement, I immediately sent him a few compositions. That same evening, my phone rang. It was Michael, inviting me to perform my songs at a charity gala in the south of France.

One concert leads to another, and everything quickly falls into place. I started out alone with just a guitar in the taverns of northern France, eventually earning invitations to small festivals, and then finding myself as the headliner. I soon realized I needed to form a band because larger stages demanded more than an acoustic setup. Press reviews were glowing, concerts piled up, and my schedule overflowed with interviews and live performances on local radio stations. The audience was always there, and for the first time in my life, I felt like my career was truly taking off. I had never been so happy!

I have so many anecdotes to share... Like the time I stopped a train because I had forgotten my guitar onboard, or the night I sang a cappella in a packed open-air theater after a storm caused a power outage. I teared up as an entire audience sang "Happy Birthday, Lili" in unison. I spent over two hours after a concert signing autographs and taking photos, or the day Alex, sitting in the car, said excitedly, "Mom, your song *Storm* is playing on the radio—how cool is that?" Writing and composing songs for Michael Jones, which he had the immense pleasure of arranging, singing alongside talented artists, performing an impromptu concert through the speakers of a TGV train after a breakdown, hosting a daily radio show during a festival, composing a song live using three random words as a challenge, and giving a concert in front of Paris City Hall. These moments were priceless.

Of course, there were also some disheartening experiences. Hearing a record label executive say, "If you looked a bit more like Dolly Parton, it would sell better..." Signing with a publisher who did absolutely nothing and having to fight tooth and nail to regain the rights to my own songs. Paying a press agent who fell far short of the experience and connections he'd boasted about. I naively underestimated the marketing side of the industry, learning tough lessons along the way.

In addition to my career as an artist, I embarked on a path as an art therapist, working with children with autism. Meanwhile, my company, Music&Motion, continued to diversify. I began offering English lessons through music in schools and hosting personal development conferences across France on the theme *"Uniqueness is a gift."* I felt fulfilled, living my passions fully while savoring the satisfaction of knowing I was making a difference every single day.

Music therapy played a crucial role in my healing journey. As evidenced by bone flutes unearthed in Germany in 2008, music has been a companion to humanity for at least 40,000 years. Long before humans invented drawing or instruments, the voice served as a tool of expression and communication. Across the globe, from Aboriginal peoples in Australia to African tribes, singing and music have been integral to rituals of prayer, celebration, and enduring hardship. Music elevates the soul, enabling detachment from material concerns. Plato, in antiquity, even reflected on the power of singing through the myth of the cicadas, describing how the Muses gifted humans the joy of song—so intoxicating that they could forget to eat.

I had the immense privilege of performing at the renowned Théâtre Sébastopol in Lille with the cast of *Zaïa*, a musical that brings together artists from *Les Papillons blancs*, an association dedicated to supporting children with mental disabilities and their families. These extraordinary artists harness their intuition to express themselves through dance and singing, often reclaiming confidence shaken by societal prejudices.

Art follows no rules; it transcends logic and rationality. Instinctively, these performers reach deep within themselves to convey emotions, sharing them with both the audience and fellow artists. On stage, we experienced a profound sense of communion. The barriers that often divide us dissolved, replaced by the unifying power of art, creating a collective experience that was as unforgettable as it was transformative.

Writing songs and sharing them with the public has been the most profound therapy for me over the past few years. My hypersensitivity, once a burden, finally found its purpose and a way to express itself meaningfully.

I vividly remember the day I wrote the song *Apology*. During one of my art therapy sessions, a mother with terminal cancer shared her heartfelt wish. She expressed her desire for her husband to find a new companion quickly, someone who could become a loving and caring mother to their two young children. Her love for him was so deep and selfless that she wished for him to move forward and not remain tethered to the past after she was gone.

Her words, embodying a love that transcended even her own mortality, shook me to my core. It was a moment that captured the essence of what it means to love unconditionally, inspiring me to channel that raw, powerful emotion into music.

You don't have to see all the tears in my eyes,
But just set me free with a sweet good bye,
Flying away and writing my last song,
Though you were the one I waited for so long, so long

And all through the years, the weeks, and the days,
You knew I had to, really had to leave someday,
There's nothing else, and nothing else that we can say.

Then, during the lunch break, I finalized the music. *Apology* felt like it wasn't something I wrote but something that wrote itself—as if my emotions were dictating the words. That day, the amphitheater was packed. Exams were looming, and group projects were being organized, but my friends understood I wouldn't be joining them. My mind was elsewhere. All night, I had thought about that mom, her gaze piercing me. Every time I closed my eyes, it returned. Sleep was elusive.

I recall a fascinating experience during a music therapy workshop involving a patient and a therapist, each wearing headsets with sensors. This process, known as hyperscan, allows researchers to observe interactions on a neurological level. During the session, the patient's brain activity shifted dramatically from processing deeply negative emotions to a sudden peak of positive feelings. Shortly afterward, the therapist's hyperscan reflected the same change. (Aalbers et al., *Music therapy for depression,* CDSR, 2017.) By analyzing the frontal lobes—the brain's emotional processing hub—scientists documented synchronization between the patient and therapist, a phenomenon in music therapy known as coalescence.

I've personally felt this powerful emotional connection many times, especially in my work with children with autism. The association *Écoute ton cœur* (*Listen to Your Heart*) will always hold a special place in mine. They were among the first to trust me. These moments of music therapy seemed as beneficial for the children as for their parents, who would relax and enjoy coffee together in the next room while I worked with their little ones.

Each session lasted 45 minutes with a group of four or five children. The first few meetings were challenging—some were afraid, others hesitant to participate—but over time, an intimate bond formed. They began to see me as *Lili,* someone they looked forward to meeting every Saturday morning.

I want to take this moment to send a big kiss to Joséphine, now twenty-two, whose iron will and strong spirit have led her toward a bright future. It's moments like these that remind me how transformative and meaningful these connections can be.

What caused this change? Music, simply. By implementing active music therapy techniques, I encouraged creativity in a dynamic and engaging way. Depending on their age, the children participated in vocal, rhythmic, or instrumental workshops, and some even composed their own music or songs. "In emergency rooms, artistic activities (music, crafts, clown interventions, etc.) help reduce anxiety levels, fight against chronic pain, and lower blood pressure, especially in children, but also in their parents," as noted by the World Health Organization (WHO).

One of my fondest memories as an art therapist was my time in the operating room at Lille University Hospital in 2012, where I discovered that music could act as a sensory bridge. While I didn't fully understand the mind-body connection then as I do now, seeing the smiles on my young patients' faces was proof enough of its power.

Here's an excerpt from my research, which gave me the opportunity to observe the mind-body connection from two unique perspectives: first, as a therapist-researcher in the pediatric surgery operating room, and later, as someone navigating the complexities of chronic pain:

"Art therapy allows the child to approach the passage to the operating room in a different way. It is one of the most valuable therapeutic approaches in managing pain in children and anticipating anxious pain. Music creates a reassuring cocoon. The pleasure of acting comes from the pleasure of accomplishing oneself, allowing the child to maintain their active status and fostering social bonding."[*]

Music not only offers an emotional escape but also becomes a tool for resilience, enabling children and their families to find comfort during challenging medical experiences.

The profession of art therapist is truly magical. Despite moments of frustration, the small, daily victories are precious and irreplaceable. Children with autism, who often have altered social and cognitive abilities, tend to respond more positively to musical stimuli than other forms of communication. Music captures their attention and holds their focus for longer periods. Improvised music therapy can even elicit "joyful" behaviors, "emotional synchronicity," and "initiation to engagement" in these children. [1]

I have so many moving stories that showcase the incredible mechanisms of music therapy in action. One story, in particular, perfectly illustrates its transformative power.

Little Matthéo had an intense aversion to *"A Sky Full of Stars,"* a song by Coldplay that, at the time, was playing constantly on the radio. The song triggered extreme anxiety in him, and his parents couldn't understand why. When his mother learned that this song was part of the end-of-year show, she was convinced her son could not participate. She feared it would provoke a crisis similar to one he had recently experienced in a store, ruining the celebration for everyone.

But what happened at the show was nothing short of magical. The

---

[*] (*Lili Road, L'Art-thérapie à dominante musicale au sein du bloc opératoire de chirurgie et orthopédie de l'enfant, op. cit.*)

photos captured Matthéo's radiant joy as he danced, sang, and played the tambourine on stage in front of a full audience and his ecstatic parents.

This moment was a profound testament to the healing power of music. It didn't just change Matthéo's experience of the song—it allowed him to reclaim a part of himself, overcoming a deep-seated fear through connection, rhythm, and joy.

A miracle? Not at all.

This transformation is due to the scientifically proven therapeutic virtues of music therapy. The fundamental principle of this approach is to reprogram the brain by replacing negative responses to stressful or painful situations with positive ones. This shift improves our emotional state and our reactions to specific triggers.

In Matthéo's case, his initial negative mental and emotional association with the Coldplay song was gradually replaced with a positive one during our sessions. What began as a negative anchor was transformed into a comforting sensory experience. Through consistent effort, we worked together to turn the song into a reassuring musical interlude—a safe and welcoming space for Matthéo.

Music therapy offered him an alternative perspective: the song was no longer associated with "stress" (undesirable emotions and behaviors) but became linked to "song and dance" (positive emotions and behaviors).

The result? On the day of the show, Matthéo not only embraced the music but also managed to express his emotions freely and connect with the world around him. It was a profound example of how music therapy can unlock doors that once seemed firmly closed.

CHAPTER TWENTY-SIX

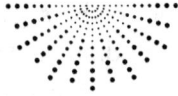

On this June morning in 2023, as I sit at my desk, bathed in the soft glow of the rising sun, I feel compelled to darken the otherwise promising outlook of summer by addressing the weighty topic of relapses. Chronic pain, like an ever-present shadow, looms over me, a sword of Damocles reminding me to remain vigilant, never fully at ease.

My first relapses, back in November 2022, were a brutal reminder of this reality. It felt as though the nightmare had returned with renewed ferocity. Like Bill Murray in *Groundhog Day*, I found myself caught in an unbearable time loop—living the same pain over and over again, day after day, week after week.

Companion as we roam, doubts in numbers call it
    home.

Just when I begin to believe I am making meaningful progress on my healing journey, the symptoms return, creeping back into my nights to disrupt my sleep, and slowly seeping into my days. Before long, it feels as if the back pain has grown worse than before the surgery. I am terrified, ensnared in a negative spiral I cannot escape. Envisioning any kind of future feels impossible.

It was a tumultuous time for my relationship. My mood swung wildly between bursts of joy for life and plunges into profound darkness. At times, life seemed to regain a sense of normalcy, strengthened by the bonds that held us together. Yet, other times, an inevitable emptiness crept in, threatening to unravel the fragile equilibrium.

As a teacher, I've come to accept a hard truth: the healing curve— learning not to feel pain—follows the same rules as any learning process. It is rarely linear, and relapses are a natural part of the journey. The path to recovery requires unlearning deeply ingrained patterns and reprogramming my brain. This process unfolds in three distinct phases.

Plateaus, for instance, are crucial moments of stasis, during which my brain forms zero pain connections. Though they feel like stagnation, these periods are pivotal. It is during these plateaus that my brain learns to release its grip on fear and stop triggering unwarranted pain responses. The stillness of the plateau is a training ground for letting go.

Recognizing this, I must remain motivated and steadfast, working with the same enthusiasm, even when progress seems imperceptible. Patience is not just a virtue here—it is a necessity.

* * *

Relapses are normal, common, and even inevitable on the path to healing. To reestablish healthy habits, my brain must first relinquish the bad ones it has clung to for so long. This transitional phase creates a kind of chaos—old habits begin to fade, but the new connections are not yet solidified, allowing pain and confusion to take root in my body.

During a relapse, symptoms may shift, intensify, or even morph into new ones. Trust me, I've experienced my fair share of these episodes: being unable to move, lie down, or sleep due to unbearable pain. Then there were periods of intestinal distress and the unwelcome return of migraines.

During one particularly difficult crisis, I found solace by revisiting an old love—the piano. While searching online for sheet music, I came across a quote by Kenny Werner, a renowned American pianist known for teaching the emotional and spiritual benefits of music: **"Don't quit a day before the miracle happens."** I immediately jotted it down in my "life journal." That simple line reignited my motivation. After twenty years away from the keys, I thought, *Why not start playing again?* It became my anchor during relapse phases—a reminder that the best was still to come.

When the final phase, the progression phase, begins, it feels like emerging into the light after a long, dark tunnel. My efforts finally bear fruit. I successfully reprogram the dysfunctional alarm system in my brain, and I can redirect my energy to the activities that bring me joy and fulfillment. My mind settles, and the rhythms of normal life begin to return.

So, how does a relapse actually work? Imagine listening to the same song on repeat for months until it becomes imprinted on your memory. It's like creating a hit! Have you ever heard a song on the radio that you didn't like initially, but after hearing it repeatedly, you found yourself humming it in the shower? Now imagine that *song* is fear.

When I try to change the playlist—replacing *The Anthem of Fear* with *The Ode to Safety*—my brain, ever cautious, clings to the familiar. It gravitates toward what it knows best, replaying the tragic duet of fear and pain. Even if the new safety melody begins to play softly in the background, my brain resists. It hesitates, doubts, and refuses to listen.

But the key is persistence. Just as a new song eventually grows on us with repetition, so too can the melody of safety take root—if I keep playing it long enough. Gradually, it replaces the old refrain, creating a harmony that my brain can finally embrace. And that's where the true healing begins.

Listening to two songs simultaneously creates a cacophony in the brain—and this cacophony represents a relapse. As we try to shift our thoughts and reactions to stress, we essentially rewrite our brain's chemistry. That's why symptoms can change so unpredictably: they may vary in intensity, appear or vanish suddenly, or even migrate within the body. These fluctuations test my enthusiasm and determination. At this crossroads, I face two choices: continue reprogramming my brain with safety messages or surrender to fear. The latter would reinforce the pain pathway, eventually transforming it into a four-lane highway. My brain would then endlessly replay the same painful melody: "Ouch, ouch, ouch, ouch, ouch...!"

But I refuse to let fear dominate. Fear only has as much power as I grant it. Instead, I take a step back and remind my brain: "I know what you're up to! Don't bother—I won't give in to fear or panic anymore!" The most intense relapses have always occurred precisely when I was on the verge of breaking free from the fear-pain cycle. They were not failures but proof of progress—signals that I was on the right neural path. That's why I call these episodes the "last honorable stand of pain."

Burrhus Skinner, a renowned Harvard psychologist, argued that our behavior is deeply conditioned by our environment. Whoever or whatever controls the environment also controls us. Skinner famously demonstrated this through experiments that showcased the power of conditioning. In one remarkable study, he taught pigeons to play ping-pong by using a reward system, motivating them to perform increasingly complex actions in exchange for food. In another experiment, he placed a rat in a transparent box with a lever. At first, pressing the lever provided food consistently. Later, the food distribution became random, and often the rat received nothing. Confused and anxious, the rat frantically pressed the lever with increasing aggression until it ultimately gave up.

This experiment reminds me of how my brain behaves when pain dominates. Like the rat, it fixates on patterns and habits that no longer serve me, frantically reinforcing the old pain pathway. But just as the rat's environment could be changed to improve its behavior, I can also recondition my brain. I remind myself that I am not powerless in this cycle. I can rewrite the story. By actively choosing new behaviors, sending safety messages to my brain, and anchoring myself in the present moment, I can move beyond the chaos of relapse and into the peace of progress.

It's a bit like my daughter and her two-year-old tantrums, the terrible twos. When a crisis erupts because I didn't choose the right pair of shoes or the right color of spoon, she cries, screams, and gets angry... Imagine the scene! The crisis reaches its climax, and then what happens? If I don't react, the tension subsides, and I hear a small voice say, "Mommy, I want a [snack or toy]." A peak of excitement and irritation occurs because my daughter, like the rodent, understands that her behavior no longer serves any purpose: the rodent's need to eat or my daughter's need to wear pink sandals in the winter. This is exactly what happens with my pains.

My brain has been conditioned to produce pain, so that's what it does. The behavior persists as long as it is reinforced: as long as the rat hopes for food, it persists in pressing the lever. As long as my little one thinks she is winning the battle, she cries. As long as I'm afraid, I hurt. When I no longer let my brain drag me into its game and no longer fear pain, it then attempts a last honorable stand before finally resigning to leave me in peace. Pain has been an integral part of my life for so long that my brain has almost become addicted to it. It will not give up overnight without a struggle.

At this moment, brain plasticity is not in my favor. Pain has become so entrenched that it has become an automatic response, while zero-pain neural pathways have weakened over time. Thus, to heal, I must accept relapses for what they are: a normal step in the process. If I try to heal at all costs, I am only delaying my recovery.

* * *

"Do I really want to heal?" This shocking question may leave you perplexed. Yet, I found myself asking it. It is scientifically proven: experiencing pain undoubtedly offers certain benefits of which we are unaware. Following F. Skinner's work, behaviorists have shown that any behavior can be shaped, modified, diminished, or reinforced by manipulating the direct environment. W. E. Fordyce was one of the first to apply this model to pain, showing that acute pain can become chronic due to the behavior of the environment (family, friends, colleagues, healthcare professionals, etc.). Indeed, consciously or unconsciously, we benefit from secondary gains that pain provides: a more involved spouse in managing children and household chores, changes in working conditions, more attentive children, or a neighbor offering help.

Secondary gains refer to all these positive side effects of pain, and the fear of losing them is sometimes a cause of relapse. Ceasing to suffer means the end of certain privileges. No more, "Can you do the shopping, dear? I have too much back pain to move," or "Can you take care of the little one tonight? I'm hurting all over!" or "I have a terrible migraine again; can you take my place at the meeting, please? I'll owe you one!" You'll agree; it's always pleasant to be pampered and to feel cared for, even if, unfortunately, it's due to our pains. It's hard to admit, but it's true. When others see us suffer, they are more considerate, offer help they never offered when everything was fine, inquire about our well-being, and give us more attention. Pain then becomes almost an identity.

Moreover, not hurting anymore means no more excuses. It implies returning to the frantic pace of exhausting and sometimes unrewarding work. It's returning to the super mom/dad fast-paced life, where only what you don't do is pointed out. Finally, chronic pains offer time for oneself and rest, even if it's forced. In short, pain is an undeniable excuse to lighten one's schedule in all areas.

This phenomenon can be completely unconscious, and even if these benefits are not entirely the cause of the pain, they can contribute to its chronicity. Thus, even though at first glance I did not feel concerned, I still took the time to think about it honestly without outright rejecting this possibility. If you are currently suffering or are with someone who is suffering, consider it without shame. The idea is not to judge or blame oneself, only to better understand oneself to heal better or help a loved one heal. That's why it is essential to know how to face the "crutches" that secondary gains can be.

After searching for a miracle cure all my life, it only took me six months to overcome my chronic lower back pain thanks to the MBC method. Some people, once they understand the causes of their pain, manage to overcome it in a few weeks; others will take years to find their salvation. Indeed, not hurting anymore or playing the piano is, in both cases, a new score for our brain.

CHAPTER TWENTY-SEVEN

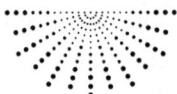

"If you are resentful, you are constantly sending yourself the message that you have been hurt. Such thoughts are perceived by the body as a huge source of stress. [...] What a relief to realize that forgiveness first has beneficial effects on ourselves, and that the main reward we get is the reappropriation of the power we have over our own lives. Forgiving certainly does not mean forgetting the offense, excusing bad behavior, or obliging reconciliation. Forgiving is, above all, giving ourselves the chance to move from the status of victim to the hero of our own existence. As selfish as it may seem, forgiving is doing ourselves good, not the other." *(Luskin, Forgive for Good: A Proven Prescription for Health and Happiness, Harper One, 2002.)*

Research in neuroscience has revealed that forgiveness is linked to a complex neuronal mechanism, and it is now proven that forgiving reduces the intensity of chronic pain. To reprogram my brain, I realized that I needed to forgive—to cut the energetic cord tethering me to the past. Retaliation, I learned, offers only fleeting satisfaction and never truly breaks the cycle of harm.

On May 24, 2023, I hear on the radio that Tina Turner has passed away. A great woman who inspired me to become an artist, Tina's strength and resilience have always been a source of immense admiration. On this somber occasion, I choose to share on Instagram a quote of hers that profoundly shaped my perspective:

> *"I do not forgive to excuse the wrongs others have done to me. I forgive people so that they no longer have power over me."*

Unresolved negative emotions are stored in our bodies, leading to the production of additional stress hormones. At best, resentment and bitterness create general discomfort; at worst, they manifest as repressed anger and chronic pain. Conversely, forgiveness is a choice to break free from the toxic cycle of anger, hatred, and psychological suffering. By refusing to waste my precious energy on resentment that silently corrodes me, I have chosen to liberate myself from the weight of the past and the destructive thoughts that consume me. This freedom allows me to savor the supreme pleasure of peace in the here and now. Forgiveness is undeniably challenging, but it is profoundly redemptive.

* * *

Ho'oponopono, an ancient Hawaiian practice passed down orally for generations, embodies this philosophy. The term *ho'oponopono* translates to "to set things right." Traditionally, it was a ritual of forgiveness and reconciliation used to restore harmony within the community. Recognized as a "living treasure" in Hawaii's constitution in 1993, its simplicity has made it a popular tool in family therapy in the West. Its playful and meditative nature lends itself well to teaching forgiveness and mindfulness—even to children.

I introduced this practice to my youngest daughter as a way to navigate her "terrible twos" with love and understanding. Together, we repeat four words, like a mantra, in moments of tension.

- **"Sorry"**: We acknowledge our emotions and the impact of our actions.
- **"Forgive me"**: We mutually offer and seek forgiveness for what has just occurred.
- **"I love you"**: We reaffirm our bond with words and a hug, placing love at the center of our relationship.
- **"Thank you"**: We express gratitude, closing the ritual with a sense of peace and reconciliation.

This simple practice doesn't solve every problem, but it's a powerful way to "reset the counters." Emily now releases her negative emotions more easily, and her tantrums are shorter and less intense. For me, these moments of post-crisis cuddles have become transformative. They allow me to let go of the emotional weight such tense episodes generate.

As a mom, facing an inconsolable child can feel like an emotional storm—helplessness and guilt swirl together. Through *ho'oponopono*, I've learned to anchor myself in love and gratitude, creating a space where both Emily and I can find peace and reconnect.

* * *

Forgiveness is not about excusing or forgetting the wrongs committed against us. Nor does it mean remaining silent about offenses or letting them go unchallenged. Forgiveness does not exclude the pursuit of justice, the need for accountability, or the boundaries we set for our well-being. It does not require reconciliation unless both parties desire it. At its core, forgiveness is not a gift we give to others—it is a profound act of self-compassion. The offense may have existed, but as Kolinka, an author and concentration camp survivor, aptly said, *"We are not obliged to live with it."* (RTL Matin, 27/02/2023).

Forgiveness means choosing the emotions we wish to feel and deciding how much power the harm done to us will continue to wield over our lives. It is a deliberate decision to reframe the way we perceive the one who hurt us—not to justify or condone their actions, but to prevent our own suffering from becoming perpetual. Forgiveness acknowledges that a person's essence may hold more weight than their mistakes. Importantly, forgiveness is a unilateral choice: we can forgive someone who does not admit guilt, who remains unreachable, or who has passed away. The process does not depend on their acknowledgment or participation.

Contrary to the belief that forgiveness is a sign of weakness, it demands great courage. To forgive requires releasing the tightly held grip of anger, the craving for revenge, the ache of injustice, and the weight of sadness. Resentment ties us to the past, keeping the wounds fresh and our freedom constrained. Choosing to forgive is choosing to reclaim our present and liberate our future.

In my own journey toward forgiveness, I've explored techniques to help me in this transformative process. Anchoring myself in the present and grounding in my breath have been essential tools. When resentment or anger begins to surface, I pause, take a deep breath, and remind myself, *"I am here and now. I no longer need to be connected to this painful past. Everything is fine now. I can enjoy my life and be happy."*

With time and self-reflection, I've begun to assess past hurts with greater honesty and kindness. Am I entirely without fault? Or have I, too, been unpleasant, reactive, or hurtful at times? When I honestly confront my own fallibility, I am reminded that I, too, am human. The old proverb holds true: we often see the speck in someone else's eye but miss the beam in our own. This recognition humbles me, guiding me to release the bitterness and desire for vengeance that poison the spirit.

To forgive is a choice. It is a conscious decision not to nourish resentment or let bitterness take root. Forgiveness allows us to sever the chains of pain and live fully in the present. It is a choice only we can make for ourselves—and in making it, we give ourselves the ultimate gift: *freedom*.

For some past events, I found it necessary to clarify what truly happened. By using expressive writing techniques, especially dialogue, I could evaluate whether my perspective on the event aligned with objective reality. This step sometimes revealed surprising truths—it helped me see if I had misinterpreted or exaggerated the situation. Was the offense as severe as I initially thought? Could it have been a trivial misunderstanding or an overreaction on my part? Often, pride prevents us from revisiting such instances. We cling to our version of events, reluctant to admit we might have overreacted or misread the situation.

With time, and a measure of wisdom earned through experience, forgiving has become easier. I've come to understand that life offers endless opportunities to feel slighted or offended, but to live peacefully, I must consciously choose to let go. Forgiveness does not signify weakness; it is a strength. Letting small things slide elevates me above my emotions, making me the master of them. A stranger cut ahead of me in line—so what? Are two stolen minutes worth the stress and negativity? A friend forgot about a lunch we'd planned weeks in advance—does this single oversight deserve to overshadow decades of friendship?

The ultimate step in forgiveness is learning to feel compassion. A person's actions are often "an expression of love or a cry for help."* This perspective reshapes my understanding of others. Happy people rarely cause harm. When I remember this, compassion naturally follows. It allows me to see that people are not fundamentally malicious—they are human, like me. Perhaps they are suffering, overwhelmed, or battling their own inner demons.

When we hurt others, whether mentally or physically, it often stems from the pain we carry within ourselves. In *The Mastery of Love*, Don Miguel Ruiz beautifully illustrates this idea: if we could see someone's emotional body as clearly as their physical body, we would notice it is skinned, covered with wounds, scars, and injuries—just like ours. Recognizing this shared humanity transforms judgment into understanding and resentment into compassion.

Behind these doors... What tales do they enfold?
Behind these doors... If walls their whispers told?
Behind these doors... What mysteries unfold?
Behind these doors...

---

* (Marianne Williamson, Facebook post, 25/10/2011)

I've always appreciated the humorous wisdom of Robin Williams, who once remarked, *"Anyone who thinks they can't change the past has not yet written their memoirs."* He had a gift for delivering profound insights with levity and charm. Often, we put unnecessary pressure on ourselves by comparing our lives to the seemingly perfect snapshots of super moms, extraordinary spouses, and ultra-performing colleagues. Yet, these comparisons are seldom rooted in objective reality. Perhaps it's time we gave ourselves a little grace and embraced our imperfections.

As I wrote this section, I found myself yearning for real-life examples of forgiveness—proof that it's not just possible but transformative. I needed to see that others had done it so I could believe, *"If they could, why not me?"* In my search, I discovered incredible stories of resilience and forgiveness, and I felt deeply grateful for these beacons of hope. Their examples serve as reminders whenever I'm tempted to lose my temper over trivial matters. One name that frequently appears on my gratitude list is Kim Phuc, whose remarkable story continues to inspire me.

Nick Ut's iconic photograph of Kim Phuc running naked down a road in Vietnam is seared into the collective memory of humanity. Taken in 1972, the image captures the aftermath of a napalm attack on the village of Trang Bang, carried out by an American unit under the command of Captain J. Plummer. The strike, described as targeting enemy forces, left innocent civilians like Kim with devastating injuries. Horribly burned, she spent 14 months hovering between life and death, enduring 17 excruciating surgeries. Today, her body still bears the scars of that horrific day.

In 1996, as a UN Ambassador, Kim spoke at a ceremony commemorating the end of the Vietnam War. She concluded her speech with these powerful words: *"If I could find the man who gave the order to drop the bomb, I would say this: 'We cannot change history, but we can now try to do our best to defend peace.'"*

What happened next was extraordinary. A man approached her and quietly said, *"I am that man."* It was J. Plummer, the very person who had authorized the napalm attack. Wracked with guilt, he had left the military the day after the bombing and devoted his life to ministry as a pastor. Without hesitation, Kim took him in her arms and said, *"I forgive you, I forgive you."*

* * *

On May 13, 1981, in St. Peter's Square, Pope John Paul II was struck by three bullets fired at close range by Mehmet Ali Agca. Gravely injured, it took months for him to recover. Yet, just days after the attack, on May 17, 1981, the Pope publicly forgave his assailant. On December 27, 1983, he went further, visiting Agca in Rebibbia Prison, fifteen kilometers from the Vatican. During their private conversation, they spoke about the secret of Fatima and what the Pope saw as his miraculous survival. Afterward, he declared: *"Today, I was able to meet my assailant and reiterate my forgiveness, as I did immediately, as soon as I could. We met as men and as brothers."*

Similarly, on January 28, 2018, sixteen-year-old Christine's life changed forever. Crossing Bab Touma Square in Damascus with her friends, she was caught in a rain of hundreds of shells. Seriously injured, Christine lost a leg and found herself in the hospital. Yet, despite the immense physical and emotional pain, she said: *"I couldn't help but smile despite all the pain and start praying to God that I would be the last victim of these mortars and that He would forgive them for their deeds... If we do not forgive, we cannot live with others."*

Another extraordinary example is that of Maïti Girtanner. Arrested at age 21 by the Gestapo for her work in the French Resistance, Maïti endured brutal torture at the hands of a young Nazi doctor, who inflicted methodical blows to the base of her spine, leaving her body irreparably damaged. She survived by a miracle in February 1944 but bore lifelong pain and was forced to abandon her dreams of a career as a pianist. Yet, despite this harrowing experience, she felt an overwhelming desire to forgive. In 1984, Maïti met her torturer and extended forgiveness with a grace that can only be described as heroic. Reflecting on her life, she said: *"I understood that a life is not measured by the projects we set for ourselves or the ideas we have of ourselves, but by the way we face the circumstances imposed on us."*

These stories illustrate a profound truth: without forgiveness, happiness remains elusive. Peace begins within us. Research shows that 70% of individuals suffering from chronic pain experience anger towards themselves. (Okifuji et al., *"Anger in chronic pain: investigations of anger targets and intensity," Journal of Psychosomatic Research*, 1999.) I've felt this anger too—the gnawing resentment, the shame, the guilt. But none of these emotions serve me. I am not responsible for what has happened to me, and I refuse to let these feelings paralyze my healing.

Today, I choose to make peace with myself, to let go of anger, and to release the heavy burdens of shame and guilt. I deserve joy, fulfillment, and the best that life has to offer. As Maïti, Christine, and Pope John Paul II remind us, peace begins within. By choosing forgiveness, we unshackle ourselves from the chains of bitterness and open the door to healing and happiness.

When my career began to take off, an ironic twist of fate presented itself: the very people who had caused me so much pain as a teenager sent me friend requests on Facebook. The turnaround was surreal—those who had shown no interest in knowing me during high school now sought to publicly display a connection to me on social media.

I won't lie and say I agonized over the decision for long; I didn't. I knew I didn't want revenge, nor did I want to continue carrying the weight of resentment. As I reflected further, I realized that the wounds they inflicted had, in part, shaped my creativity, inspiring some of my most heartfelt songs. In an odd way, those experiences, however painful, contributed to my journey and my art.

So, I accepted their invitations. But we never addressed what had happened in the past. No apologies were exchanged, no deep conversations took place—it didn't feel necessary. The power those memories once held over me had already faded, replaced by a sense of closure I hadn't anticipated.

Today, twenty-five years later, I can definitively say that chapter is closed. It no longer stirs the same hurt or anger. It's simply a part of my story, one that I've made peace with—and for that, I'm grateful.

CHAPTER TWENTY-EIGHT

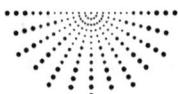

*F*reed from a burden, I can now focus on calming my brain by rebuilding good daily habits. My two primary areas of focus: sleep and nutrition.

During the darkest period of my life, I longed for a peaceful night —a night without insomnia, pain, rumination, or waking in the middle of the night to take pills. Pain is always worse at night. The intense feeling of loneliness amplifies everything. The memory of one particular night before my emergency admission to the clinic remains vividly etched in my mind. I was in crisis, lying in the middle of the living room, crying and groaning. I just wanted everything to stop.

That night, the house felt frozen in time, plunged into a state of shock. The next day, my little one was awake, demanding my attention, but the pain was stronger than me. I screamed—I couldn't help it. It hurt too much. I couldn't even lie down anymore. At the height of despair, I called emergency services. I broke down in tears on the phone with a doctor:

"I can't do anything more for you, Madam. You'll have to wait. There's no point in going to the emergency room—it's too crowded. You're already on the highest levels of morphine and painkillers... I'm sorry. Call your surgeon tomorrow."

I thought morning would never come.

Sleep is not a straight line. It consists of successive cycles. According to Inserm, a good night's sleep comprises three to five cycles of about ninety minutes each. To feel rested in the morning, you must reach the phases of deep sleep, where the body recovers most effectively from physical fatigue accumulated during the day. During this phase, the entire body is at rest while the brain stores energy for the next day. Dreams, on the other hand, occur during REM sleep, a phase where the muscles remain inactive, but the brain is highly active.

Scientists believe dreams serve two essential functions: to process and convert daily experiences into useful lessons for the future, and to anticipate challenges to better prepare for them. Unfortunately, my sleep cycles are so fragmented that the quality of my sleep is poor, preventing my body from recovering properly. The extreme fatigue I feel the next day lowers my pain tolerance and intensifies the emotional strain. This disturbed sleep also fails to play its restorative role in the healing process, further complicating my recovery.

But the vicious cycle doesn't stop there. To get through the day, I allow myself a nap, but if it extends too long, I struggle to fall asleep at night. Even when I resist napping, exhaustion doesn't guarantee rest. I often find it impossible to get comfortable enough to fall asleep, and in those moments, I'm tempted to take a sleeping pill. If I resist, pain often acts as an alarm clock, waking me repeatedly throughout the night.

At 5:00 a.m., the radio still plays the night's news, and even the rooster hasn't crowed yet. Still, my day of pain begins. Exhausted, I feel trapped, less active, and unable to effectively manage my pain. I move less and turn to food for comfort, deepening the trap. It's a massive spider's web, and I am stuck.

However, since sleep quality has a profound and rapid influence on chronic pain, improving it must become an essential part of my self-care plan. Dr. Hanscom, an American orthopedic surgeon, attributes at least 25% to 30% of his patients' recoveries to better sleep quality. This gives me a simple yet powerful tool to enhance my physical and mental well-being.

The billions of cells in our brains are constantly communicating, generating subtle electrical currents known as brain waves, which vary in frequency depending on our activities. At bedtime, while still awake, our brains produce beta waves—those associated with everyday activities and alertness. To transition to sleep, however, the brain needs to slow down and emit alpha waves, which occur in a state of calmness, relaxation, and serenity. These waves help chase away stress, anxiety, and other mental noise that disrupts rest.

The challenge arises when thoughts loop endlessly in my mind. The more I replay yesterday's events or worry about tomorrow, the harder it becomes to shift out of beta waves and into the relaxed state needed for sleep. Counting sheep doesn't work because my brain remains stuck in overdrive. Intrusive, negative thoughts can make the situation worse: *"The perfect mom at the parent meeting looked so zen. She even took notes to write a report. I'm so useless..."*

The key to countering these destructive mental loops is to reestablish healthy habits. First, I will modify my lifestyle with simple but effective changes. Then, I'll tackle the "sleep thieves" in my environment and regain control over the stimuli that disrupt my rest. Acquiring good sleep habits, practicing relaxation techniques, and cultivating positive thoughts will help me fall asleep more easily and improve the quality of my sleep.

* * *

Home Sweet Home. Today is a big day—I'm finally returning to my room. After months of enduring a medicalized mattress on the living room floor, followed by convalescence in a medical bed upstairs, I've decided it's time to reclaim my cozy big bed beside my sweetheart. I've had enough of mattresses as hard as bricks. I can't wait to dream again of sunny beaches, with the colorful shadows from my bedside lamp dancing across my beautiful surfboard hanging on the wall. And more than anything, I'm looking forward to my little one snuggling between her Daddy and me for morning cuddles once more.

Similarly, I will tackle the insomnia fueled by my overactive creativity and endless to-do lists. If, like me, you tend to jot down tomorrow's plans while in bed, I strongly recommend stopping.

Instead, I've decided to make my lists before dinner, giving my brain plenty of time to process them well before bedtime. On my bedside table, I've placed a pretty pink "life notebook" and a pencil—not for tasks, but for gratitude. At the end of the day, I'll write down the things I'm thankful for. And if a stray thought insists on lingering, I'll jot it down and promise myself to deal with it tomorrow.

I'm also learning to respect my biological rhythm while adapting to my little early riser. Since her birth, she's often awake by 5:45 a.m. While that's perfect for grabbing fresh croissants (or pain au chocolat, if you prefer!), it's less ideal for maintaining energy all day. So now, whenever I feel the first signs of fatigue—no matter what I'm doing—I'll head to bed. Sticking to a regular bedtime is crucial for establishing long-term good sleep habits. These days, I even set an alarm to wake a little before my daughter, which sometimes gives me the luxury of meditating in peace before her day begins.

With the intensification of my physiotherapy sessions, physical exhaustion helps me fall asleep more quickly. However, if I find myself ruminating, tossing, and turning in bed, I've learned not to fight it. After half an hour, I'll get up for a glass of water or a comforting hot drink, meditate, or dive into a good book—resisting the magnetic pull of social media. To give the sandman every chance, I only return to bed once I've calmed my mind and slowed down my metabolism. And I've made a firm decision: no more naps. Instead, I opt for relaxation techniques to recharge, which I'll share with you soon.

Another change I've embraced is moving my evening mealtime two to three hours earlier, giving my body time to transition toward rest. I've also established an evening ritual to signal that bedtime is near—something I had always ensured for my little ones but neglected for myself. The biggest trap? Scrolling through social media. Why? Everything we see or hear in the hour before bed has a higher chance of infiltrating our dreams and nightmares. So, I replaced mindless scrolling with a gratitude practice, a gentle way to prepare for restorative sleep.

Returning to my own bed has also done wonders for my relationship with Cam. Pain had taken up so much space in our lives that it created distance, straining our bond. Watching a loved one suffer without the ability to ease their pain is deeply distressing—it can leave one feeling helpless and, at times, even rejected. But something as simple as holding hands can rebuild that bridge. Research shows that empathetic touch, like holding hands, synchronizes breathing, heart rate, and even brain waves with those of a partner. (Goldstein et al., "Brain-to-brain coupling during handholding is associated with pain reduction," *PNAS*, 2018.) This connection fosters understanding and support while activating the brain's natural pain-relieving mechanisms.

Another simple yet powerful ritual? A relaxing massage before bed. Not only does it temporarily reduce pain and promote sleep, but it also strengthens the bond within a couple. A secure relationship creates a secure and peaceful brain. For far too long, our intimacy was over-shadowed by pain—an uninvited third party in our relationship. It was always Cam, my pain, and me. But now, we've evicted that "intruder." The mood in our bedroom is one of warmth, music, candlelight, and sensuality. Between us, there's no longer any room for pain—only the promise of rediscovered connection and shared joy. My sweetheart, my faithful accomplice in this journey, supports me in every way possible. Together, we are reclaiming the life we deserve.

A mindfulness meditation, self-hypnosis, a **prāṇāyāma** exercise (Sanskrit for "breathing"), yoga nidrā, or even a touch of music—thanks to advances in neuroscience, I've added new techniques to my toolbox to relax, calm my nervous system, and gently shift my thoughts away from pain. Each evening, I choose my favorite method to help guide me toward the calming alpha wave state.

Tonight, I settle in comfortably and select a visualization exercise, crafting a soothing mental image. I hear the rhythmic roar of ocean waves, their whispers lulling me into serenity.

Symphony of water whispers what it yearns to sing.

I feel the warmth of soft sand beneath my feet and the cool embrace of an evening breeze on my face. When an unwelcome thought intrudes, I don't resist it. Instead, I acknowledge it, become aware of it, and gently return my focus to my bodily sensations. With every inhale, I steady my mind. With every exhale, I release tension.

My breath becomes my anchor, grounding me in the present and silencing the echoes of anxiety about potential insomnia.

Gradually, I feel my pulse slow, my body cool, and my awareness root itself in the here and now. The waves continue to sing their gentle melody.

Sweet dreams.

CHAPTER TWENTY-NINE

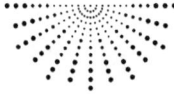

When I face stress or discomfort, I often find myself turning to food for solace. In these moments, my choices are less about nourishment and more about "eating my emotions."

Now, let's take a closer look at what happens in our intestines during such moments. Every time we eat, we're not just fueling our bodies—we're also feeding trillions of microbes that inhabit our gut. These microbes play a critical role in our overall health, and scientists are discovering new ones every day. Think of our digestive system as the body's energy factory. For this factory to operate efficiently and deliver high-quality fuel to our cells, we need to nourish the "right workers"—the favorable microbes that act as allies to our health.

For example, when I eat vegetables rich in natural fibers, I'm feeding the beneficial microbes that protect against chronic pain, heart disease, and inflammation. On the other hand, the unfavorable microbes thrive on sugar. When I give in to an impulse and reach for processed cookies, these harmful microbes flourish, promoting inflammation and slowing the body's natural healing mechanisms. Making mindful food choices sends a powerful message to my brain: *I have value, I care for myself, my body has value, and I am taking care of it.*

One simple rule for healthier eating is to "eat a rainbow." The vibrant colors of fruits and vegetables come from phytonutrients—natural compounds that plants use to protect themselves against germs, insects, and the sun's effects. While not essential like vitamins or minerals, these phytonutrients help prevent certain diseases and support overall bodily function. Unfortunately, the typical Western diet, often described as "beige," lacks this variety of colors, as it tends to prioritize heavily processed foods over fresh fruits, vegetables, and natural antioxidants.

Studies illustrate this starkly. When mice are fed a Western diet, they exhibit increased inflammation, nerve hypersensitivity, and an overactive immune response. These mice also heal more slowly, experience prolonged pain, and show notable weight and fat gain. (Christ et al., "Western diet and the immune system: an inflammatory connection," *Cell*, 2019.)

The winning combination? Vegetables, fruits, and whole grains. A colorful, balanced diet feeds the good microbes in our gut, promoting stability and diversity in gut flora. Research consistently shows that this type of diet reduces inflammation and alleviates pain in individuals with conditions like fibromyalgia, migraines, rheumatoid arthritis, osteoarthritis, and musculoskeletal pain.

To support my healing, adopting fresh and varied foods is essential. However, a healthy and balanced diet isn't a quick fix; the changes must be sustainable to truly impact our health. Ideally, half of our plate should include whole grains rich in natural fibers and antioxidants, such as whole-grain bread, pasta, and brown rice. The other half should primarily consist of colorful seasonal vegetables and fruits, celebrated for their antioxidants and anti-inflammatory properties.

Adding to this foundation, healthy proteins like fish, poultry, eggs, legumes, and nuts are vital, along with the use of healthy oils such as olive oil, walnut oil, flaxseed oil, or chia oil in place of butter or cream. To preserve nutrients, cooking food at low temperatures is recommended. Conversely, it's important to limit the intake of red meat, dairy products, added sugars, and processed foods, all of which are linked to higher inflammation levels.

For a little sweetness, I use natural alternatives in moderation, such as stevia, maple syrup (a loving nod to Canada!), agave syrup, kitul sap, and honey. These not only replace white sugar but also add unique flavors to the homemade cakes I love baking with Emily and Mathilde. Another secret weapon in my pantry is brewer's yeast. It's a power-house of benefits—strengthening the immune system, promoting healthy hair and nails, fighting bloating, regenerating intestinal flora, and being rich in protein. During my pregnancies, brewer's yeast became an essential ally, thanks to its high vitamin B9 content, crucial for fetal development.

Vitamin D also plays a significant role in well-being. Over 50% of Americans are deficient in vitamin D, despite its importance for overall health. Exposure to sunlight, regular physical activity, and maintaining a stable, healthy weight can help boost this vital nutrient. *

Now that I'm back at the family table, cooking together has become a source of joy. For the sake of our health, our figures, and our taste buds, we've made significant changes to our diet, including dras-tically reducing red meat. My gentleman-cook is now a regular in the kitchen, enthusiastically preparing dishes with chicken, fish, and vegetables straight from our city garden.

Though our urban garden is much smaller than the one we once had in the countryside, it still brings us together. Emily reigns as the queen of the pink watering can, diligently tending to her lettuce, tomatoes, and spinach. Yet, her true delight lies in plucking ripe rasp-berries straight from the bush and savoring them on the spot.

To prepare for summer and achieve a healthy tan, dietary supple-ments can be helpful, but a carrot juice cleanse before the season begins is another fantastic option—a little trick passed down from my mother and grandmother. Nourishing our bodies with fresh, nutrient-rich foods is one of the greatest gifts we can give ourselves. This natural medicine comes without side effects and helps us savor life to the fullest. It's no wonder that people suffering from chronic pain often struggle with maintaining a balanced diet.

The usual culprits? Lack of time, fatigue, and a never-ending to-do list. The lunch break? Often postponed until I realize it's closer to

---

* https://my.clevelandclinic.org/health/diseases/15050-vitamin-d-vitamin-d-deficiency.

snack time. Yet meals should be cherished as rituals—moments to care for ourselves and to connect, whether with friends, family, or colleagues. Shared meals foster essential socialization for every generation, from the youngest to the oldest.

In France, we've recently embraced the Nutri-Score system to help guide our food choices during shopping. This label rates products from A to E, with Nutri-Score A (dark green) representing the most nutritionally favorable items and Nutri-Score E (red) indicating less favorable options. However, it's important to note that a D or E rating doesn't necessarily mean a product is unhealthy. For instance, olive oil, despite its many health benefits, is rated C due to its high caloric density. This is because the Nutri-Score is calculated per 100g of a product, not per serving. While consuming 100g of pasta in a meal is realistic, consuming 100g of oil is far less likely. Thus, the Nutri-Score is most effective when used as a comparative tool within a balanced diet. For example, at the same price, should I choose brand X lasagna with a Nutri-Score of C or brand Y with a Nutri-Score of E? Similarly, it can help resolve daily dilemmas, like Emily's choice between caramel cream and yogurt—her two favorite desserts.

Hydration is another cornerstone of well-being. When you feel thirsty, it's already too late! A study highlights the significant benefits of staying hydrated, particularly for managing pain. Researchers at Massey University in New Zealand examined healthy men aged 22 to 32. On the first day, participants drank their usual amount of liquids. On the second day, they abstained from drinking for 24 hours. Afterward, both groups underwent the same pain resistance test: immersing their feet in ice-cold water for four minutes. The results were striking. Dehydrated participants couldn't tolerate the cold water for as long, showed signs of hyperventilation, and experienced an accelerated respiratory rate and reduced blood flow to the brain.

The takeaway is clear: eating well is essential, but drinking (water!) is just as critical. Hydration directly influences our ability to manage discomfort and maintain overall health. Whether you're healthy or dealing with chronic pain, never underestimate the power of a well-hydrated body.

* * *

In our societies, food often intertwines with emotions and sociability. Don't we celebrate milestones and cherished moments with a "good meal"? Yet, when I turn to food to soothe my emotions, I am merely numbing them with comforting choices—the infamous "comfort foods." Curiously, I never attempt to soothe discomfort with a piece of fruit. Emotional eating usually involves foods rich in sugars and saturated fats, which trigger an immediate release of dopamine. It's a fleeting burst of pleasure often shadowed by a pang of guilt.

Why the guilt? Because emotional eating doesn't satisfy a physiological hunger; it addresses a psychological void tied to physical or emotional suffering. I eat without hunger, seeking solace or release. A cookie becomes a placeholder for emotional emptiness, chips absorb my frustration, and candy becomes a vessel for guilt.

A critical tool for managing chronic pain and resisting the pull of emotional eating is **mindfulness.** By observing and accepting my bodily sensations, I can decipher their true nature. Is it hunger, signaled by physical cues like a growling stomach or muscle tension? Or is it a compulsion—a desire to snack without genuine need? If it's the latter, I dig deeper to identify the underlying conditioning.

Pop culture, for instance, plays its role. Shows like *Friends*, which I adored, have embedded the trope of drowning sorrows in pints of ice cream. So, when I feel the urge to binge, I ask myself: Am I tired? Do I hurt? Am I lonely or overwhelmed by emotions or stress? Once I identify the trigger, I take a step back and focus on my breathing.

When the craving looms, I ground myself in the present and ask aloud, "Do I really need to eat this pack of cookies? Is this what I truly want?" Instead of fighting my emotions, I allow them to surface. I acknowledge them with kindness and without judgment. Rather than reacting impulsively, I redirect my brain toward a healthier comfort: I meditate, sip tea, chew sugar-free gum, or use my "call a friend" lifeline. By offering my brain an alternative "madeleine de Proust," I create new associations and pathways to soothe myself.

Questing for all, content with none,

Seize it, but joy swiftly gone.
When in your hands what you wanted,
It's already lost appeal.

Never being fully connected to what we are doing or eating contributes significantly to losing touch with our physiological cues. When we multitask—eating while watching a video, for example—our brain struggles to process both activities effectively. Is it focused on eating or watching? To counter this, I now avoid eating in front of my computer, TV, or, even worse, my mobile phone. Instead, I use meal-time as an opportunity to talk, relax, or enjoy something auditory, like a podcast, a radio show, or music. I also make it a point to put down my utensils between each bite, allowing myself to savor the experience fully.

Cam and I are finally rediscovering our daily routines and reestablishing our good habits. We delight in preparing vibrant, rainbow-colored dishes that are a feast for both the eyes and the palate. Using a variety of spices, we engage all our senses, slowing down to truly appreciate the experience. I focus on the taste of each bite, observing the moment food meets my tongue, and consciously listening to my sensations. Internally, I describe the colors, flavors, and aromas of what I'm tasting.

Drawing inspiration from tea meditation, I create what I call "the plate of life." A colorful table spread, the aroma of fresh ingredients reaching our nostrils, and the joy of a burst of flavors dancing on our tongues—these small details bring satisfaction to both my senses and my mind. This mindful approach to eating transforms a simple meal into a deeply enriching experience.

CHAPTER THIRTY

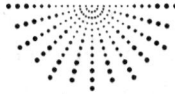

*W*ith over three hundred concerts per year in my schedule, I spent countless hours on trains. Enveloped in music, I often found myself mesmerized by the rhythmic dance of landscapes rolling by. These moments of quiet reflection, suspended in time, became my sanctuary. I often shared photos of these fleeting scenes, capturing the serenity they brought me before the energy of the stage. Have you ever taken a long detour home because you missed a highway exit—not because you were distracted, but because your mind had wandered elsewhere? Or found yourself so absorbed in thought that the world around you faded away? These experiences capture the essence of a hypnotic trance—an altered state of consciousness we all naturally enter multiple times a day. Far from being a rare phenomenon, these moments are vital for maintaining our mental balance.

While the term "hypnosis" is relatively modern, its mechanisms date back to ancient times and are increasingly reclaiming their place in therapeutic care. As Dr. Lorenzi-Pernot explains, "Medical hypnosis is not what you see on television, where a snap of the fingers places someone entirely under another's control. It is a normal physiological state... which the brain enters approximately every eighty minutes during the day in adults, often without us realizing it. The idea of hypnosis is to harness this natural ability."*

Whether managing my chronic pain, improving my sleep, or regaining control over my eating habits, hypnosis has enabled me to tap into previously untapped inner resources. Our unconscious mind governs approximately 85% of our overall functioning, effortlessly handling a variety of complex tasks such as reading, driving, or playing sports. Additionally, it serves as the archive of all our experiences, both positive and negative. However, the conscious and unconscious parts of our minds do not communicate directly.

This disconnect explains why, even if I consciously remind myself, "Food is not the solution to stress," my unconscious might still follow a deeply ingrained program that equates stress with raiding the cookie jar. Until the unconscious recognizes that new suggestions are beneficial, it resists change. Hypnosis bridges this gap. By inducing a trance state, the conscious mind becomes saturated, allowing the unconscious to accept positive suggestions and replace harmful behaviors or negative mental patterns.

Self-hypnosis, in particular, creates a space for personal transformation. In this state, I can reorganize limiting beliefs and reprogram my unconscious mind. You don't need unwavering self-confidence to begin; action itself fosters confidence. Initially, self-hypnosis might seem daunting or evoke apprehension, but these fears are entirely unfounded. The day I realized this, it felt like a revelation—a genuine "wow" moment.

Have you ever tested your receptivity to hypnosis? You might discover, as I did, an openness within you waiting to be explored. Since practicing self-hypnosis, I've significantly reduced—and nearly eliminated—my episodes of binge eating, and insomnia no longer plagues me. It isn't a miracle cure, but once you master the basics, it becomes an incredibly effective tool.

As Milton Erickson wisely said: "Trust your unconscious. It's a

---

* Dr Lorenzi-Pernot, sep-ensemble.fr/traitements-parcours-de-soin/auto-hypnose-douleurs, 2014.)

wonderful way to live, a lovely way to get things done... Don't try to use someone else's technique. Just discover your own." *

Only you know where your doubts will roam
Only you know where your road finds home

For instance, when it's time to fall asleep, I no longer need a full hypnosis session. With practice, my brain has become so familiar with the scripts I've created that a simple countdown paired with a suggestion is enough. I rarely even reach the number 20 before drifting off. Here's how it goes:

"You're sleepy, you yawn. In 30 minutes, you fall asleep. You're tired, you want to sleep. In 29 minutes, you fall asleep. You're tired from your day, you feel exhausted. In 28 minutes... Sweet dreams!"

---

* Erickson et Courtis, *Le sens vibratoire et les acouphènes, musique et hypnose, Revue française de musicothérapie*, 2017.

CHAPTER THIRTY-ONE

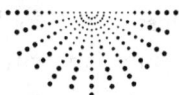

Sixty thousand! On average, we have sixty thousand thoughts per day, turning our brains into a bustling anthill. But it's crucial to pay attention to this ant invasion! A staggering 80% of this swarm consists of "ANTs": Automatic Negative Thoughts. These are the thoughts that ruin our days and haunt our nights. Interestingly, we are only aware of 10% to 15% of our thoughts, and over 95% of them are identical to those of the previous day. Since our brain doesn't distinguish between what benefits us and what harms us, constantly dwelling on negative thoughts leads us to believe them, shaping them into our reality. That's why I must become the vigilant "guardian" of my own thoughts! (Robins quoting his mentor Jim Rohn, *The Jim Rohn Guide to Personal Development,* Success, 2014.)

Many things to oversee,
I'm overwhelmed, can't you see?
And they've taken up so much space,
Sharpen your blade for this chase.

Buddha explains that painful events are like being struck by an arrow, posing the profound question: "If you are struck by an arrow, will you shoot another arrow at yourself?" To illustrate this teaching, he shares the story of a man who, after being hit by an arrow, becomes consumed by anger and rumination, adding layers of psychological pain to his physical suffering. Through this metaphor, Buddha emphasizes that our interpretation and reaction to events—not the events themselves—determine our happiness or unhappiness. Pain is inevitable, but suffering is optional.

Consider the frustrations of everyday life: stalled home improvement projects (perhaps professionals would've been a wiser choice!), endless traffic jams (who came up with this new traffic flow on Becquart Avenue?), or the lingering "terrible twos" of a seven-year-old (isn't this supposed to be the age of reason?).

These challenges are the first arrow: inevitable and universal—this is life! But we can avoid shooting the second arrow, the one we inflict upon ourselves through blame—"Of course, they always dump the worst files on me!"—self-pity—"Why does this stuff always happen to me?"—or misguided coping strategies—"Chocolate... or gummy bears?" This second arrow keeps the wound fresh, preventing it from becoming just another scar in the tapestry of life.

To leave that arrow in its quiver, I must choose to accept what happens to me—everything that happens to me. But let's be clear: "acceptance" does not mean "passivity." On the contrary, it calls for deliberate action. Acceptance is the foundation of resilience, a refusal to let circumstances define us. It's a choice to move forward, scars and all, with strength and grace.

Our brain functions much like a computer, continuously compiling and archiving the information it receives. If I program it negatively, the output is predictably negative. This is why my immediate responses to triggers are often not conscious decisions but conditioned reflexes. Automatic thought mechanisms, deeply tied to our personality traits, play a significant role in how our nervous system reacts to daily stressors. To thrive, it's essential to find balance—to leverage our traits without becoming overwhelmed by their adverse effects.

For a long time, I believed the pressures I faced were mostly external. However, research shows that individuals who objectively reflect on their experiences of burnout often acknowledge that much of the pressure comes from within. Chronic pain and burnout share a striking commonality: a hyper-demanding nature toward oneself.

It's hard to imagine a life entirely free of stress. Neither you nor I can stop working or performing daily tasks. But we can reimagine a life where stress no longer dictates our mental and physical suffering— a life where we manage daily challenges calmly and with grace.

I invite you to join me in a transformative thought challenge. Let's defy our automatic thoughts together. Starting today, we will replace self-criticism with resilient, constructive, and forward-looking perspectives. When life tests us, we will focus on solutions rather than getting trapped in rumination.

Mindfully, I encourage you to observe challenging situations with kindness, without judgment or filters. This practice will teach you how to rebuild your thought patterns into ones that are nuanced and empowering. I now refuse to remain imprisoned by the whirlwind of negative thoughts that serve no purpose other than to harm my mental and physical well-being.

When I catch myself spiraling into negativity, I interrupt the cycle with a firm and audible, "STOP!" I then take a deep breath and intentionally shift my focus to the positive. Acceptance means calmly acknowledging the entirety of a stressful situation and considering rational solutions. It does not mean passivity—it is a choice to face life head-on.

I've also learned to confront my emotions as they arise, rather than suppressing them and allowing them to fester in my unconscious as emotional parasites. Trust me, your life will transform the day you become aware of the second arrow you shoot at yourself. It has been a long journey of personal development for me, but when your life philosophy changes, everything changes.

CHAPTER THIRTY-TWO

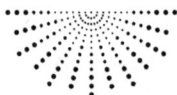

*t's possible that, like me a few years ago, you believe breathing is an automatic process and that our bodies naturally breathe correctly. Learning to sing and discovering *prāṇāyāma* (breath control) proved to me that this is not the case. As a concerned young mother, I often tiptoed into my little ones' rooms to ensure they were sleeping well. With babies, it's easy: I would remain silent and watch their tiny bellies inflate and deflate. Phew! Everything is fine! I now know that babies instinctively practice what is referred to as "sacred breathing"—a complete abdominal breath that is foundational in the yogic tradition.

Unfortunately, as adults, we often adopt bad habits that lead to tension and anxiety. Accumulating stress and suppressing emotions shifts us from complete, regular abdominal breathing to irregular, shallow thoracic breathing that fails to engage the abdomen. Take a moment to observe your own breath. Do your shoulders rise? Yes? Does your belly inflate? No? If so, you're practicing thoracic breathing, and your lungs are likely only filled to 30% of their capacity.

Thanks to singing, I had some experience with abdominal breathing, but it wasn't yet automatic for me. More recently, through yoga, I discovered techniques to deepen and enhance this practice. Breathing and well-being are closely linked: an agitated state of mind leads to chaotic breathing, while a calm state of mind produces steady, peaceful breaths. Proper breathing improves our physiological, psychological, and energetic states, which is why I feel immediate relief whenever I focus on my breath.

The term *prāṇāyāma*, formed from *prāṇā* (breath) and *yāma* (control), refers to "the cessation of disturbances in breathing" or the art of circulating universal vital energy (*prāṇa*) throughout the body. This concept extends beyond the biological function of breathing, encompassing a "movement of life" with profound effects on health, mindset, and self-awareness. Deep, complete breathing forms the foundation of meditation, yoga, relaxation, and even sports. Interestingly, it's often wrongly assumed that inhalation is the most critical part of the breathing cycle. In reality, "one must always exhale more than one inhales: this way, we expel more carbon dioxide and waste than we bring oxygen to the body" (Dr. Rougier, *actinutrition.fr/themes/douleurs*).

Thus, I began practicing various breathing techniques and was fascinated by the sensations I could feel simply by altering my breath. My *prāṇāyāma* workshops focus on two main objectives: better breath control and reducing the physical and psychological impact of stress and pain.

One such practice is *mahat prāṇāyāma*, the complete three-stage breath (*mahat* means "large" or "big" in Sanskrit). It consists of three steps:

1. **Abdominal breathing:** The belly inflates as the lungs fill, pushing the diaphragm toward the navel.
2. **Thoracic breathing:** As the diaphragm contracts further, the lower ribs expand outward and forward.
3. **Clavicular breathing:** The shoulders rise as the diaphragm reaches maximum contraction.

To exhale, the process reverses: starting with the clavicular area, then the chest, and finally the abdomen. When I first practiced this technique, I found it helpful to sit upright on a chair, imagining *prāṇa* rising within me during inhalation and descending during exhalation. Through regular practice, I now sense this energy flow. If you'd like to try, focus on two key aspects: inflating your belly during inhalation and lengthening your exhalation.

This complete breathing technique allows the lungs to fill to maximum capacity, efficiently oxygenating cells and eliminating toxins responsible for stress and anxiety. Agitated, uneven, or jerky breaths signal anxiety to the body, while calm, regular breaths promote peace and relaxation. The inseparable connection between breath and mind is echoed in an ancient Taoist text: "Breath is guided by thought, and thought is guided by breath" (Tsou Lu, *Le Secret de la fleur d'or*).

Breath retention (*kumbhaka*) can be practiced in two ways, each with distinct effects:

- **Retention with full lungs** reduces physical, psychological, and energetic tension.
- **Retention with empty lungs** fosters introspection and invites a sense of letting go.

By extending exhalation, I help detoxify my body of carbon dioxide, enhancing oxygenation of the nervous system. Initially, this practice required intense focus, as the sensation of asphyxiation triggered fears of suffocation and even death. These reactions reminded me how the subconscious mind can magnify fears. Full lungs symbolize life and vitality, while empty lungs evoke vulnerability and mortality. Over time, embracing the concept of "letting go" helped me accept the duality of life and death, allowing fear to dissolve.

Have you heard of the 365 method? Developed in the United States about 15 years ago, heart coherence stems from advancements in neuroscience and neurocardiology. While one might assume the heart beats like a metronome, even in a healthy person at rest, heart rate variability is normal. This variability increases during stress and decreases during relaxation. Heart coherence helps regulate breathing to control these variations, sending calming signals to the brain. The

365 method involves three daily sessions of six breaths per minute (inhaling for five seconds, exhaling for five seconds) for five minutes.

Perhaps, like me, you've postponed these exercises, claiming you don't have time. But if I can dedicate three minutes while brushing my teeth, surely I can prioritize my brain's health alongside my dental hygiene. After all, what could be more important?

CHAPTER THIRTY-THREE

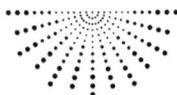

hroughout my artistic career, I have had the immense joy of serving as the godmother for several associations and dedicating my time to organizing events aimed at fundraising for medical equipment, funding foreign medical care, or supporting research into new therapies. Through this work, I have been in close contact with parents of children with severe disabilities or serious illnesses, and they have taught me invaluable lessons in resilience.

What always touches me is the immense stress, anxiety, and physical fatigue they endure daily—yet they never let themselves be defeated. To this relentless pressure is often added a heavy burden of shame and guilt, as these parents feel they can never do enough for their child. As a result, many suffer deeply, both in mind and body.

What saddens me most is that these parents often feel guilty for taking even a brief respite. When they allow themselves a single week of vacation to recharge, placing their child in an institution where they are well cared for, they judge themselves harshly. Despite dedicating three hundred and fifty-eight days a year to their child, they feel as if they are abandoning them.

Every aspect of their lives becomes a struggle: finding a place in school, financing innovative therapies, and planning for their child's future in a world where they may no longer be present. Moreover, the caregiver often becomes a bystander, their emotional well-being inextricably tied to the physical and mental state of the person they are caring for.

Too small to understand, as they say,
But then too small to suffer in this way.
Feeling so helpless, they smile,
Hopeful soul, so pure in style

"Today, Leo is having a good day. He's trying to communicate with his little sister and me. He even agreed to get dressed without complaining. And, for once, he didn't choke at the table."

"It's so difficult. Today, Leo refuses to wash, dress, or eat. He's sitting in his chair, unresponsive to any of my requests. And when I try to approach him, he tries to hit me."

The anxiety parents feel is not confined to the present moment; it extends to the future. What will happen to their child once they are gone? Who will take on the role of caregiver? Siblings?

Caring for a parent, child, spouse, or friend—whether elderly or unwell—is a profound responsibility, one that often carries a heavy emotional toll on both body and mind.

* * *

"The greatest joys come with the greatest pains." Becoming a parent is a daily challenge and, at times, a far more arduous task than one could have imagined. Goodbye to relaxing showers, sleeping in, quiet reading on the toilet, and spontaneous outings. Hello to greasy hair (maybe I'll just call it a sebum treatment), early wake-ups (the early bird catches the worm, right?), rushed bathroom breaks (forget the reading), and the supreme desire to be under the covers by 9:00 p.m. (the first bottle is due in two hours!).

Being a parent is an immense source of happiness, but it also involves a monumental lifestyle shift. Psychological and emotional stress levels rise, while time for self-care shrinks to near invisibility.

Parenting means being on high alert all day, every day. It's no coincidence that the government's 2011 campaign, "1000 First Days, Young Parents," featured a couple fretting over their crying baby: "Do you think it's normal for him to cry so much?" A few minutes later, they're asking, "Is it normal for him to sleep so much? Should we wake him up?"

This scene perfectly captures the anxiety of young parents. If the baby sleeps too much, we worry. If the baby doesn't sleep enough, we worry even more. And this concern for their well-being never ends. As the child grows, too much noise in their room makes us nervous, but no noise at all is even more alarming.

Then comes adolescence, leaving home, and eventually the role of grandparent. Parenting is exhausting on a psychological level because we will always find a new reason to worry.

Moreover, being a parent is a challenge that often leads to frustration. Reconciling "child" and "career" peacefully is no small feat. The constant juggling act between personal aspirations and parental responsibilities is a reality that all parents face.

And the emptiness of my womb, will I ever feel forgiven
And his heart locked up in a tomb, and that piece of him
  in heaven,
And no way he can face this truth as he felt so heart-
  broken.
And living through so much more, yet no tears can bring
  salvation.
And this little grain of love, this little spark of folly, too
  many words unspoken.

When a man between twenty-five and fifty visits the doctor complaining of pain that seems to have "come out of nowhere," it's often revealed that he has recently changed marital status or become a father. (Dr. Stracks, www.johnstracksmd.com). This is a delicate subject to address. Admitting to professional burnout is far easier than acknowledging parental burnout. Society makes it incredibly challenging to confess that, even momentarily, we may have regretted our role as parents. Yet, I believe we must free ourselves from such guilt. Let the parent who has never had this thought cast the first stone!

Being a parent means taking on the role of a caregiver, prioritizing the child's well-being above one's own under any circumstances. This selflessness is admirable but can also be a double-edged sword.

Paradoxically, 35% of parents—often mothers—suffer from "empty nest syndrome." (Copper-Royer, *Le Jour où les enfants s'en vont*, Paris, Albin Michel, 2014). In my case, I experienced an intensely challenging period when two waves of emotional upheaval collided:

First, I suffered from a profound melancholy tied to a sense of abandonment and emptiness after my eldest left home. No one is ever truly prepared to watch their little ones leave, especially when it feels sudden. Despite what others might say, the sadness that follows is not offset by the newfound time for self-care. I decided not to let myself become a passive victim of this transition. Slowly, I learned to treasure the little things—the brief texts and fleeting moments of joy with my children. Although I see them less now, our reunions are filled with meaning and joy, and I cherish them deeply.

Second, I struggled with postpartum depression that lingered due to challenging family circumstances. Adding to this, I had to navigate raising my youngest—a "Covid-19 baby"—who exhibits many traits associated with this unique label: heightened anxiety, difficulty managing emotions, and frequent night terrors.

Researchers have found that maternal stress and elevated cortisol levels during pregnancy significantly influence a child's ability to develop emotional regulation. (Rash et al., *Maternal cortisol during pregnancy is related to infant cardiac vagal control*, Psychoneuroendocrinology, 2015). Reflecting on this, I realize how much my own stress during those uncertain times may have affected her.

Furthermore, like all children born during this period, my youngest daughter experienced a very atypical start to life: limited outings, no visits, no family gatherings, and a profound lack of opportunities for socialization. Even experienced childminders, including one who cared for my seventeen-year-old son Alex, confirmed that children they have cared for since the end of the lockdown are noticeably more challenging to handle. These children cry more often and struggle to regulate their emotions.

I've come to realize how much my reactions have shaped my youngest daughter's beliefs and fears—particularly about pain and her ability to endure it. By adopting an attitude of acceptance, I can model resilience and effective emotional regulation for her. This realization also highlighted the importance of creating a warm and supportive atmosphere at home.

My chronic pain has undeniably affected our family dynamics. It's difficult to organize family events when the living room is dominated by a medical mattress and a constant reminder of suffering. The resulting atmosphere can feel oppressive, leading to conflict and frustration. This awareness hit me like an electric shock. We decided to break this cycle by organizing a small birthday celebration with Emily's friends to mark her third birthday. Restoring the family home to its role as a safe, joyful, and reassuring haven is crucial for her well-being.

Looking back, I realize that during my mom's migraine episodes, I often felt a deep, unconscious sadness and guilt. Seeing someone you love in pain—without any way to help—is a helpless and heartbreaking experience.

If you've seen the movie *Bohemian Rhapsody*, you may recall the Zoroastrian creed: "Good thoughts, good words, good deeds." Farrokh Bulsara, better known as Freddie Mercury, tirelessly sought his father's recognition, even as his father struggled to accept his life choices. Being a parent is never easy. It means guiding a child while respecting their individuality, offering unwavering support, and loving them unconditionally, regardless of their decisions or path in life.

None of us had perfect parents. None of us are perfect parents. And our children won't be perfect parents either. So, today, if you're a parent like me, I suggest we pause and acknowledge everything we're doing right—both the small gestures and the monumental efforts.

We achieve remarkable things every day. When our children are small, they throw tantrums. When they become teenagers, they can be ungrateful. And yet, we look back on the baby's midnight cries with tenderness, even as we sit awake waiting for a sixteen-year-old who's over an hour late. Eventually, they arrive home with a big grin and say, "You waited for me?"

It's only when we become parents ourselves that we truly understand the profound anxiety—and unparalleled joy—of parenting.

CHAPTER THIRTY-FOUR

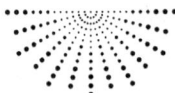

*W*e achieve dozens of small feats every day—as parents, colleagues, or friends—yet we rarely consider them true successes. Often, out of modesty, we attribute our victories to luck, circumstances, or the alignment of the stars. In reality, we have every right to proudly proclaim that we are proud of ourselves. To boost our self-esteem, we must dare to give ourselves credit. In fact, year after year, the sum of all these small successes strengthens our mental image and self-confidence. We should not deprive ourselves of that.

I have always felt that taking care of myself was unproductive and encroached on all the other tasks on my to-do list. However, now I believe that taking care of oneself must be number one on that list. Science confirms it: I cannot pour from an empty jug. Now, before worrying about the well-being of others, I will pay a little attention to my own. It's not selfishness; it's a matter of survival. I must become my first source of inspiration and enthusiasm. If I do not love and respect myself, how can others love and respect me? Establishing a well-being ritual is not superfluous; it is not wasted time—it is essential! Anything that brings relaxation, joy, and happiness must have a special place in my task lists.

When I mention the word *well-being,* I do not necessarily mean a bubble bath and scented candles. Although that is an extremely pleasant moment, it is a narrow view of the term. In reality, to be happy, I must create a true *Well-Being Bubble.* Within this introspective bubble, I can ground myself in the present when a daily challenge arises. Taking care of oneself is extremely difficult in painful periods. Why take care of a body that betrays us, hinders us in our lives, movements, and relationships with others? Why take care of this carcass that causes us pain? However, sometimes it's because our brain loves us that it makes us suffer, and that awareness is violent but effective. I will listen more carefully to my needs and desires, or else I will run straight to my physical and psychological downfall.

Creating this bubble of self-confidence and faith in the future involves a sense of gratitude. Despite the difficulties I am currently facing and the neuropathic pains I have to learn to live with, I am alive. I breathe! I have not become paralyzed! I see my children growing and flourishing, and I am very proud of them. Many would say, "How lucky you are!"

Rooster crow! In the 1920s, it was French pharmacist Émile Coué who popularized the immense power of autosuggestion. By repeating positive thoughts, I generate more positive thoughts and create a snowball effect. Do you remember the diligence and love with which *The Little Prince* took care of his rose? Now, I take on that commitment and responsibility; I will water the flower of enthusiasm in my life daily, despite the pains. I am like a caterpillar in its cocoon, and I will emerge transformed from my chrysalis. I will know my limits and accept my imperfections because no one is perfect. Moreover, I will protect myself from those who hinder progress and shield myself from toxic people by refusing to absorb their negativity, because no one is invulnerable. The grass always seems greener in the neighbor's field. Unfortunately, this quest for improvement leads only to dissatisfaction and frustration.

Best at times foes with good, you know...

Gratitude, long associated with spiritual or religious practices, puts into perspective what we really need in order to live. As rightly stated by Eli Whipp, a Pawnee Native American, to Cornelia Locke in the series *The English*: *"What you want and what you need" are two different things; all you need "fits on a horse."* Gratitude is not just a social construct, as cooperation is present in many animals who instinctively understand that the other can reciprocate. Gratitude is an adaptive trait acquired over time to promote the survival of the species. As M. de La Fontaine's King of the Animals reminds us: *"You always need someone smaller than yourself."*

The concept of gratitude may seem a bit naive, yet it is vital to our psychological balance. It encompasses a feeling of appreciation and a sense of wonder that encourage us to enjoy life. Gratitude is not limited to our "thank yous." It involves becoming aware of the positive elements we receive and recognizing that they come from an external source: be it people (family, friends, or even a perfect stranger), animals, plants, objects, or experiences, opportunities, and events. Gratitude and resilience are intimately linked because resilience finds its essence in the ability to feel compassion and love for oneself and others. This can also be found when one appreciates the small pleasures of life. It is the ability to see the positive in the negative and to sublimate sufferings into learnings, resources, or motivation to evolve.

Gratitude is all at once an emotion, a mindset, and a personality trait. It is a life philosophy that must be an integral part of our daily lives. It offers an opportunity to celebrate the present moment and be an actor in one's life. It gives meaning to the past, brings peace to the present, and creates a vision for the future. By valuing and appreciating moments for what they are worth, we focus our minds on what we have, not on what we might need: *"It is impossible to feel both envious and grateful at the same time."* (Emmons et Shelton, *Handbook of Positive Psychology*, Oxford University Press, 2002.)

I am someone who has always cultivated the "gratitude attitude"! And once again, music was often my means of expression. It's the plane of a hopeful teenager landing at Pearson Airport in Toronto, feeling that reality will far exceed her expectations. I will live a waking dream, a story worthy of a fairy tale.

The welcome in the arrival hall resembles a scene from a movie: exchange students from all over the world, members of the Rotary

Club, balloons, flowers, signs—nothing is missing. I am dropped off at my first host family. Throughout my stay, I will have several host families: all different, yet all more wonderful than the others. I am welcomed like the prodigal child; it is almost destabilizing. My host siblings and I are treated no differently in the eyes of my Canadian parents. Who could have imagined that I would celebrate my 18th birthday in Toronto and experience the transition to the new millennium in such a special place? In just a few months, I went from profound discomfort—sometimes even the desire to end it all—to a crazy desire to fully enjoy life. Everything seems possible here.

I will always remember my first day at Iona Catholic Secondary School. I had dreamed of it, and the Rotary Club made it happen. I am very proud to wear my school's uniform: a green and blue Scottish kilt, bottle green tights, a crisp white blouse, and a sleeveless green vest embroidered with the school's logo. I love it! The debate about uniforms often arises in France, but I must admit that I only saw advantages. First and foremost, I felt a real sense of belonging. And, to my great delight, I was finally not judged for my clothes. It was one less stress. As for the need to differentiate myself, it was still possible during numerous extracurricular activities and casual days.

Although enrolled in high school, I also take the opportunity to attend some university classes. The atmosphere is completely different when you are the *Frenchie* and no longer the intellectual of the group! Also, as this year will not be counted in my French curriculum, I indulge myself: singing, dancing, acting, English literature, guitar, geography, and Canadian economics classes. I want to flourish in what I love most (music) and discover this country that has always inspired me—thanks in part to my idol at the time, Bryan Adams, whom I will have the pleasure of meeting during my stay.

With *King Lear* in hand, I finally understand all the subtleties of this book. I had started reading Shakespeare's plays at home, but at that time, without the internet, it was absolutely impossible for me to grasp all the nuances. My first literature class is a real cultural shock. The teacher doesn't need to beg students to volunteer to go to the board or make an oral presentation. Here, they almost jostle each other to share their thoughts and ideas. I am obviously in a good school, but not all students come from privileged backgrounds—far from it. "Putting on a show" simply seems to be part of their DNA.

Thus, here, I can finally be myself. Entrepreneurship is also one of the favorite activities at school, as evidenced by the numerous clubs managed by the students themselves. So, I join the music club, where we organize concerts and musicals throughout the year to raise funds for charitable associations. The entrepreneurial spirit does not prevent a sense of community. I am amazed at the quality of the events they organize. At home, at that time, such initiatives were usually tackled in higher education.

Another cultural shock: my friends drive and work alongside their studies. I will even do a little internship at a florist with Wendy, one of my best friends. Both on stage and behind the scenes, I feel useful, I take pleasure, I blossom, and I learn so much. Every day, when I get on the yellow school bus—you know, the one from *Forrest Gump*—I feel so grateful! The seats are uncomfortable, the bus creaks, but it's my daily moment of gratitude. I cherish everything that happens to me while admiring the sunrise behind the CN Tower.

Wanna tell my story, wanna sing my story,
No chances in life, no mere lottery.

My schedule is like that of a minister, with each week bringing its share of surprises. Memories rush through my head as I write these lines. I feel the intense emotion of singing the Canadian national anthem, *"O Canada,"* at national events and slipping into the role of Madame de Pompadour to sing *"La Marseillaise"* with a philharmonic orchestra. I relive the excitement of Halloween, dressed as Minnie Mouse, going door-to-door trick-or-treating for candy on the streets of Mississauga. I also cherish the magic of Christmas and its traditions, which I share with families of different religious denominations.

Like a sleigh in the starlit sky,
Hanging by stars, dashing so high.
In the Christmas night's embrace,
Love's magic, such a timeless grace.

I also remember impactful experiences such as outreach in Toronto with the Scott Mission and organizing charity events with the Rotary Club. Finally, I will never forget the unique privilege of contemplating the majestic Niagara Falls through the four seasons and even sleeping in a tiny quinzhee, a snow shelter of Native American origin that resembles an igloo but is made from a pile of hardened snow. I have experienced so much, some of which I had forgotten and rediscovered when my parents dropped off boxes from my childhood bedroom.

One day, during my Canadian economics class, I heard about the Forum for Young Canadians, a weeklong program at Parliament in Ottawa designed to teach participants about Canadian governmental processes. Since Canadian citizenship was required, I had no reason to believe my application would succeed, but I decided to give it a try. To my great surprise, a few days later, I received a call from the organizers. They had been considering inviting foreign students for several years to promote cultural exchange, and I had arrived at just the right moment —I would be the first! They were even more delighted that I was French and spoke both official languages of Canada.

Being behind the scenes of Parliament was an extraordinarily enriching experience. It also allowed me to compare it with the organization of the National Assembly in France, where, as an elementary school student, I had won a contest that opened similar doors for me. I quickly found my place as a translator, a role I greatly enjoyed and fully embraced. I was frequently asked to interpret the Canadian anthem in its bilingual version to inaugurate evenings or meetings. The stay concluded with an award ceremony where I had the honor of receiving the Canadian Social Fabric Medal from the Minister of Industry, an award recognizing the promotion of bilingualism. Years later, whenever I wear this pin, I am filled with pride and joy. It even brought me luck for the *agrégation*.

I also participated in a business and international diplomacy seminar in Chicago. Even then, we were already discussing the future of the planet and global warming. Finally, I took part in a live-action role-playing game in Montreal organized by the UN. For a week, we were cut off from the outside world, self-sufficient, and fully immersed in our roles as diplomats. Day and night, we received dispatches—

diplomacy does not wait! I even began to wonder if politics might be a career for me.

Finally, I must mention my wonderful journey across Canada! I traveled from one ocean to another—two buses, about a hundred students, and over a hundred nationalities represented. We drove for miles, often with nothing on the right and nothing on the left, yet we were always amazed by the breathtaking landscapes and the sight of bears with their cubs crossing the road ahead of us. From battling mosquitoes in Winnipeg to admiring the vibrant flowers of Victoria Island and singing at the Calgary Stampede, each experience was unforgettable. Whether we slept in our sleeping bags at night or stayed with host families, these moments left me with a lifetime of cherished memories. Regardless of nationality or religion, we were united by an idealistic view of life, carrying a shared message of tolerance.

At that time, no one was absorbed by their mobile phone; we lived in the moment without worrying about crafting the perfect reel for Instagram. At each stop, we staged singing, dancing, and theater performances to thank our hosts. The essence of this trip was the "gratitude attitude." We had all experienced an incredible year, and we wanted to show our appreciation to those who made it happen. Writing this testimony, I realize how much I experienced in just one year, and how profoundly it changed the course of my life—it moves me deeply.

When the first symptoms of chronic pain appeared, it became difficult for me to cultivate the "gratitude attitude" that once defined me. Pain invaded every part of my being—body and soul. I felt like a stranger to this battered body and this flavorless life. I desperately awaited the disappearance of my symptoms to be happy. Ironically, it was precisely when I moved furthest from gratitude that I needed it the most.

Studies are clear: practicing gratitude activates the body's internal pharmacy and can help reduce chronic pain. Gratitude also plays a crucial role in rewiring the brain, fostering positive thinking, and stimulating the production of happiness hormones like serotonin and dopamine, which bring real physical, emotional, psychological, and social well-being.

Gratitude also boosts resilience. It has tangible physiological effects: it increases good cholesterol, lowers bad cholesterol, regulates blood pressure, and harmonizes the nervous system by improving heart coherence and reducing inflammation. It reduces the risks of depression, anxiety, and addiction. For example, gratitude has proven to be a key factor in suicide prevention: writing gratitude letters reduces feelings of helplessness in 88% of suicidal individuals and increases optimism in 94% of them. (Emmons, ibid.)

Spirituality transcends the religious dimension of the word. It is a personal quest for meaning in our existence—a deep desire to understand the life we lead, regardless of belief or religious attachment. This quest for spirituality and wisdom is a vast topic, too philosophical to fully explore here. However, there are simple universal keys to achieving it:

- Practice gratitude every day.
- Engage in mindfulness meditation.
- Forgive others, but also yourself.
- Engage in activities that bring joy and peace.
- Listen more, speak less.
- Stay away from troublemakers.
- Observe nature and the world with benevolence.

Adopting gratitude involves embracing a whole new mindset. I won't lie—it wasn't easy. Living twenty-four hours a day with chronic pain, the "gratitude attitude" did not naturally impose itself on me. However, I began by acknowledging the small things that brought me happiness. As Daniel Defoe wrote in *Robinson Crusoe* (1719): *"All our torments about what we lack seem to me to stem from a lack of gratitude for what we have."*

Thus, I relearned to say thank you—not the automatic thank-you of everyday life, but a heartfelt one. I became more present in my gratitude, accompanying my thank-yous with a smile, a gesture, or a look. And in doing so, I reaped far more than I sowed. Each day, I asked myself: What am I grateful for today? The presence of a loved one, a shared moment, a personal achievement, a gift, a discovery, a smile, a delicious meal, good news, a phone call, or an evening with my partner—none of these are trivial.

I also tested many gratitude workshops, and I encourage you to establish a "gratitude habit." The results are truly spectacular! It's about seeing the glass half full, every day, rather than half empty. Take three moments in your day to STOP. Clear your mind and choose one reason to be happy. Imagine your life without some of the people or things you might take for granted. Notice the little joys: a morning coffee, a ray of sunshine.

Try the ABC of gratitudes: Find something or someone starting with "A" to be grateful for today, then "B" the next day, and so on. When you've gone through the alphabet, start over!

"I love myself!"

Choose a quality, skill, or action you are proud of. From your talents to the color of your eyes, you deserve self-love. I especially enjoy reading a book with my daughter, where the heroine transforms into various creatures yet proudly declares on every page: *"I love myself, I am happy to be me!"* What a precious message to share with our children.

Although it may not be September 21 (World Gratitude Day since 1965), it's always the right time to celebrate gratitude. I want to take this moment to thank you, the reader. I thought of you while writing this book, and I sincerely hope it brings you as much emotion, hope, and happiness as I experienced while creating it. From the bottom of my heart: thank you. Writing this book gave me a reason to fight, to get up every morning, to not give up.

Don't give up, don't look back, straighten up,
keep in track and just keep pushin' on.
Although it's hard on the way, your heart and soul are
strong.

CHAPTER THIRTY-FIVE

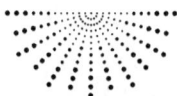

I'm reaching the end of the tunnel and, as William Ernest Henley wrote, *"I am the master of my fate, I am the captain of my soul."* This brief excerpt from Henley's poem, written while he was on a hospital bed after a foot amputation, resonates with me today as a cry of resilience. It is also the poem *Invictus* that Nelson Mandela drew strength from during the 27 years he spent in prison, fighting for civil rights. Even though I now have to deal with neuropathic pain in my foot, I no longer suffer from back pain in everyday life. It is high time I restore greatness to my life so that the pains become insignificant.

My life took a sudden turn when chronic pain appeared. Everything became challenging, both physically and mentally. I thought I had to take it easy, so I stuck to the bare minimum. The paradox? I no longer traveled, but I spent an hour in traffic to go to work. I didn't go out with my friends anymore, but I subjected myself to the Saturday "big shopping" with an overflowing cart. I no longer engaged in sports, yet I performed the exact same movements during exhausting chores. And during the remaining rest periods, I suffered, ruminated, and cried about my life and my broken body. Happiness disappeared from my radar.

The decision to "take it easy," though sensible on paper and supported by the majority, led me straight to disaster. Removing the pressure relief valves prevented my brain from externalizing the daily overflow of emotions. I became unable to clear my mind. Everything I didn't release, I kept, reinforcing the vicious circle of fear and pain.

Writing this section, I realized that chronic pain had stolen one of the most characteristic aspects of my personality: my unwavering smile. It was often mentioned in press articles when I was an artist: *"Her original compositions were as well-received as her smile and kindness," "With a big smile and humility in tow," "Lili Road radiates her energy and smile."(Le Dauphiné libéré, La Voix du Nord, La Dépêche du Midi.)*

With pain, my life became serious, and I rarely smiled anymore. I lost that carefree part and that "hopeless romantic" side that once defined me. To recognize myself again, there is only one solution: I must embark on a quest for positive emotions and double down on the "gratitude attitude."

Just a smile can go a long way.

When we smile to express happiness, our bodies release substances such as endorphins and serotonin, whose positive impacts on mood and well-being are scientifically proven. These substances reduce stress levels and the intensity of perceived pain. It has even been shown that maintaining positive facial expressions helps resist stressful situations (*Marmolejo-Ramos et al., Experimental Psychology, 2020*).

I fondly remember the coach of the Marquette athletics club who used to repeat during our interval training sessions: *"But smile, darn it! You'll go faster and hurt less!"* Bless you, Raymond! Behind this little provocative phrase was actually a genuine scientific principle. Simply smiling won't lead to an immediate cure, but smiling can contribute to one.

Of course, smiling isn't the first thing I feel like doing when I'm in pain. Yet, despite the pain, I continue to engage other muscles in my body... so why not engage the muscles in my face? Now, every time pain disrupts my life, even if it feels counterintuitive, I smile so that my neurotransmitters can tell my brain that everything is fine and encourage it to draw from its internal pharmacy to reduce the intensity of the pain.

In a study at Berkeley, researchers found that those who genuinely smile experience a real sense of joy and happiness, which they convey to the people around them. Smiling is the most effective way to surround yourself with positive people. *"Optimism is a happiness magnet. If you stay positive, good things and good people will be drawn to you."* (Mary Lou Retton, *Gateways to Happiness,* WaterBrook Press, 2000.)

Are you smiling now? Not yet? Take a deep breath with me, and let's wear a big smile together. Does it seem ridiculous? Smile for a few more moments and observe your sensations.

Since the 1970s, Dr. Norman Cousins claimed that laughing for 10 minutes allowed him to enjoy two hours without chronic pain. Humorously, he stated, *"Laughing heartily is a good way to jog indoors without having to leave home!"*(Cousins, *Anatomy of an Illness, Norton & Company, 2005*).

Unexpectedly, laughter is not a new therapeutic tool. As early as the 14th century, French surgeon Henri de Mondeville used humor to distract patients from pain during surgery and throughout recovery. From the cardiovascular to the immune system, the therapeutic virtues of laughter are numerous. Laughter triggers the release of endorphins, decreases adrenaline production, and stimulates dopamine, promoting a sense of well-being.

Bedridden and with low morale, I rediscovered one of comedian Florence Foresti's most iconic sketches: *Les Mamans Calmes* (*The Calm Moms*). Her incisive humor and portrayal of parenthood managed, for a few minutes, to pull me out of my lethargy. "My two main pillars of education are: shouting, running." That satire of the perfect mom instantly made me smile, then burst into laughter. Those few moments were precious when I was in pain.

According to the French Federation of Cardiology, a child can laugh up to 400 times a day, while adults laugh only about 10 times a day. What a waste, considering the therapeutic virtues of laughter!

Now that I'm better, I can laugh again during my little one's silly moments.

If we laugh for 10 to 15 minutes a day, we induce muscular and joint relaxation that can last up to an hour. Laughter also strengthens antibodies in the body, especially in the nose and respiratory passages, increasing resistance to migraines, depression, and insomnia.

Another key to regaining a smile is to be kind and generous. Acts of generosity make me happy. Although I regularly donated blood before my last pregnancy, I haven't participated since then. I'm looking forward to donating again now that I'm no longer taking medication. Strangely, while I dislike getting my blood drawn, this sampling doesn't bother me at all.

I will also be kind and generous to myself. When one of my children, my partner, or a friend has good news, I always offer congratulations or a small gift. I will now do the same for myself. I will treat myself, guilt-free, to a café on a terrace, a shopping spree, or a square (not 10!) of dark chocolate.

The more a neural pathway is stimulated, the stronger it becomes. By smiling, I strengthen the neural pathways of happiness, joy, gratitude, and pleasure. So, why deprive myself?

"For many lives, I had worked on myself, struggled, done everything that could be done, and nothing happened. Now I understand why nothing happened. The effort itself was the barrier, the very desire to seek was the obstacle. Not that you can reach without seeking. The search is necessary, but then comes a moment when the search must be abandoned..." *(Osho, Autobiographie d'un mystique spirituellement incorrect, Albouraq éditions, 2019).*

Reading Osho's story for the first time deeply moved me. When I understood what neuroplastic pain was, I imposed a strict regimen of writing, walking, and meditating for several hours a day. I tried to eat better, sleep more… but in the end, I exhausted myself trying to figure out how to free myself from the grip of pain. Then, one day, I had *my*revelation. I was trying to heal at all costs. However, like Osho, it was when I stopped seeking that I found.

This epiphany prompted me to write and formalize the MBC method. That's when I experienced a lightning-fast improvement. My symptoms became less painful and more scattered, and relapses became less frequent. Finally, I felt like I was living again, even though neuropathic pain in my foot is now an integral part of my life. I now have all the cards in hand. I can reinvest in my life knowing that my chronic pain will no longer play a central role. Thanks to my method, I have a painkiller on hand if fear and pain ever catch up with me.

CHAPTER THIRTY-SIX

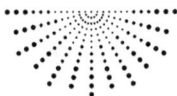

A whole new world unveils its spell,
A whole new world where dreams excel.

I have healed, just like thousands of people around the world when they discover the true nature of their suffering. It's not my desire to impose lessons with this book; I have only tried, with the help of neuroscience, to demonstrate to you that a better and pain-free world is possible. Life's trials and accidents, such as the onset of chronic pain, present an opportunity for personal development. In Chinese, the word "crisis" (weiji) is a fusion of "wei," meaning danger, and "ji," meaning opportunity. Drawing from the yin-yang philosophy, it embodies the idea that opposites—danger and opportunity—are intertwined. A crisis is not merely a challenge to overcome but also a chance to grow. Each one calls for change, introspection, and growth. They represent a true transitional tool toward a new homeostasis, with the crisis being nothing more than a tunnel leading to a new balance. It is in difficult times that we develop resilience, discover our core values, and our true identity. It is in these moments that we grow the most.

While traveling in Asia, on the way from China to India, I passed through Bangladesh, leaving me with an unforgettable memory. It seems unexpected things always happen to me. I arrived at Dhaka Airport in Bangladesh more than four hours late. We had a delayed takeoff and experienced strong turbulence throughout the flight. Since it seemed that the plane was not exactly in its prime—with some hatches quite literally held together with tape—I was already in a state of considerable stress. This flight, during which I planned to sleep to recover from accumulated fatigue, turned out to be mentally and emotionally challenging, putting my nerves to the test.

Waiting by the baggage carousel, I wait and wait for my suitcase, but no more luggage arrives. The airport is empty; it was the last flight of the day. Past midnight at the airport, I start wandering through the corridors without my suitcase and with a mobile phone that cannot find the local network. I admit that some doubts creep in. I pull myself together and, regardless of my suitcase, decide I'll deal with it tomorrow. A hotel taxi, reserved by my assistant, should be waiting for me outside the airport. Despite the delay, I trust they must have checked my flight and come back at the scheduled time. I exit the airport, but there's no one outside except for armed men. The adventurer that I was at the time keeps smiling. The heat is stifling, dust is omnipresent in the air, and I am devoured by mosquitoes and insects of all kinds. I also start to feel very thirsty.

A soldier addresses me in English: "Miss, you shouldn't stay here; it's too dangerous for you!"

"Thank you, I know that, but can you help me get to my hotel, please?"

Without even answering me, the man walks away, shrugging. Apart from sleeping in the airport lobby—it is now 3:00 a.m.—I don't know what to do.

"Miss, do you need help?" A man in a suit has just called out to me from a walkway. My savior! He introduces himself as the airport director, and, after checking his ID, I agree to follow him to his office. As for my suitcase, the news is not good; he can't locate it. As for the rest of my issues, he takes care of contacting my hotel and waiting for the taxi with me. The Radisson hotel is beautiful, with a central cathedral-like hall from which all floors can be seen. The staff pampers me; they have gathered some beautiful clothes and everything I need to freshen up. A snack is already waiting for me in my room. Despite everything, running on just two hours of sleep, I'm far from fresh when my supplier's taxi finally arrives two hours later to whisk me off to work.

All's well that ends well? Almost! I take the plane to India again, still without my suitcase. Fortunately, upon arrival, my on-site agent has prepared a small package with traditional clothes. Thanks to that lost suitcase, I had the pleasure of wearing some beautiful Indian clothes that were lent to me for a few days. If Instagram had existed at the time, I would have posted so many reels!

In India, social inequalities within the population are extremely pronounced. When I was invited to some suppliers, I discovered how little they lived with. Yet, their only wish was for me to feel comfortable. I remember being invited to a family's home that didn't even have access to running water. Despite this, they wore radiant smiles and seemed profoundly happy. Talking to them, I discovered that their philosophy of life played a significant role. They had long ago learned, without the help of self-help books, resilience. The practice of meditation was very prevalent, both among adults and children, including in schools. I found the children I encountered to be relentlessly positive and remarkably resourceful.

In my opinion, kintsugi, an ancient ancestral Japanese technique, metaphorically embodies the art of resilience. It involves repairing a broken ceramic object by highlighting its fault lines with gold powder instead of trying to conceal them. Thus, imperfections are elevated rather than masked. Chronic pain has brought my cracks to light. It battered and weakened me, taking advantage of my vulnerability to break me. However, that period is over. I have repaired each of my flaws with gold and elevated them. Thanks to them, I have become a better version of myself: stronger and more confident in the future, ready to face new challenges. Even though I still have some lingering minor pains in my back and am learning to live with my neuropathic foot pains, I am starting to rediscover my true essence. Now, I am fully intent on exploring my golden nuances. But what will I do with this new radiance?

The following statistics raise some concerns, especially when read in parallel with the reforms on the legal retirement age. Fifty-two percent of workers say they are very dissatisfied or dissatisfied with their work, and according to a very recent survey, more than 2.5 million employees are in severe burnout. (Study on Workplace Happiness Among the French, Institut Think, 2017.)

During the lockdown, and thanks to remote work (or perhaps because of it), we have all taken a step back from our professional careers. However, finding a job that we are passionate about is not an easy task. Pain forced me into a long-term sick leave, and now, I am considering a comeback. Not being happy at work can contribute to the onset of chronic conditions. Thus, as it has happened in my life before, I believe it is an opportune moment to ask myself the right questions: Does my work make sense to me? Am I in the right place? Mind you, I'm not fooled by platitudes like, "You must do what you really love in life!" which are wonderful on paper. I am well aware that life sometimes imposes decisions on us that we reluctantly make—no longer practicing the artist's profession was not a deliberate choice.

I admit that I loved being a buyer. I love to travel, and I adore human contact; it seemed like the ideal job. However, each trip left me with a bitter feeling. I had the privilege of traveling in first class and staying in celebrity suites. At the same time, I was imposing drastically low prices on my suppliers, which gave rise to a heavy sense of guilt. Emotion and business do not go well together.

So simple to shut these doors, to leave the past behind,
Yet true emotions linger, in the depths of our mind.

I formed friendships with these people, and I would have liked to contribute to improving their quality of life. Every medal has its reverse side: on one hand, I told myself that I was exploiting them; on the other, I tried to convince myself that I was helping them develop their economy. The textile companies I worked for were serious businesses, strict about working conditions, and fighting against child labor.

However, my suppliers admitted, implicitly, that they outsourced some of the work and were not always aware of what was happening with their subcontractors. Most people prefer to close their eyes to certain realities. So, upon returning from maternity leave, I seized the opportunity to request a mutual termination of the contract and funding for a skills assessment to initiate brainstorming about my professional future. It was a particularly enriching milestone aimed at understanding my true purpose in order to harmonize my personal and professional aspirations. I was ready to consider anything, including the possibility of earning less or managing my schedule differently. Therefore, after obtaining a business school diploma and holding a managerial position, reflecting on my ikigai led me to start an Art Therapy Degree at the Faculty of Medicine in Lille.

To discover what this famous ikigai is, let's continue our journey together to the Land of the Rising Sun, towards the island of Okinawa, also known as the "Island of Centenarians" because it has fifty centenarians per one hundred thousand inhabitants. In 2020, among the three thousand villagers of Ogimi, fifteen were centenarians, and one hundred seventy-one of them were over ninety years old. Like me, you may be wondering about the secret of this exceptional longevity. It is actually very simple: adopting a balanced diet (rich in green vegetables, algae, and fish, and lower in rice than the rest of Japan), engaging in daily physical activity, and above all, always having a good reason to get up in the morning. This seems to be their "magic wand."

Moreover, they claim to follow a life philosophy called ikigai. In Japanese, ikigai means "to live," but it can also be translated as "result, effect, reward." It is what drives us to get up every morning, motivates us, allows us to enjoy the present moment, and consider that life is worth living. It is a spiritual fulfillment that can be placed on the top floor of the Maslow pyramid I mentioned earlier. Ikigai is never acquired; it is not a fixed state but rather a life process in perpetual evolution. In fact, research has confirmed that those who never find their ikigai have an increased risk of early mortality. So, as our ikigai is constantly evolving, now is the opportune moment for me to reconsider mine.

* * *

First, I start with a period of introspection about everything I love to do and the activities I am good at. Then, I observe my environment and my needs, focusing on activities for which I can be financially rewarded or socially valued. Finally, I think about activities that can make a positive contribution to the world. At the intersection of these reflections, the heart of ikigai represents what gives meaning to my life, what makes me happy, and what I am meant for. In the West, the concept of ikigai has been diverted from its original philosophy, encompassing all areas of life, and is predominantly applied by coaches to the professional domain. It is then used to find jobs that align with our deep desires and values.

However, the original ikigai is an integral part of us. It is not just an activity we love to do. When we follow our ikigai, we forget the notion of time, we can move mountains, and all areas of our life are perfectly in harmony. Moreover, it nourishes us and allows us to develop our full potential. Thus, one can find their ikigai outside the sphere of work by taking care of their family or engaging in leisure activities, for example. Obviously, answering four questions is not enough to find your ikigai, and it is not done on a whim. It requires real investment and demands breaking down barriers, fears, and doubts.

In fact, while writing this book, I have the intimate conviction that the profession I currently practice will not be the last in my professional career. Resume playing music? Turn back to art therapy? Or help those suffering from chronic pain full-time? I have plenty of desires, and I will strive to consciously choose what constitutes my current ikigai.

In their book, Hector García and Francesc Miralles offer a fascinating study on the lifestyle of the centenarians of Okinawa. (*García et Miralles, Ikigai, Pocket, 2018.*) They derive ten rules of wisdom to follow to improve health and well-being, hoping to live as long and as happily as those who live according to their ikigai:

- 1 Always be active and never stop learning.

- 2 Take the time to live and approach challenges calmly.
- 3 Eat only 80% of your satiety.
- 4 Surround yourself with good friends.
- 5 Practice daily physical activity.
- 6 Smile and consider the people around you.
- 7 Reconnect with nature.
- 8 Practice gratitude and thank life for everything.
- 9 Live in the present moment.
- 10 Follow your ikigai.

So, have you thought about doing a skills assessment? Do you want to do one? It can truly be a determining step in your professional career, personal life, and healing journey. I bet you can't guess who was fired because he "lacked imagination and had no good ideas." What would have happened if Walt Disney had started brooding about being "inept in his preferred field"? What if he had given up recreating a business after each of his failures? I probably wouldn't be singing the lullaby of Ahtohallan to my daughter at night to put her to sleep (*Frozen 2*, Disney). Success is not hoping that things happen—it is putting all your enthusiasm into making them happen.

For now, my professional life will resume at Lille University while I wait to see what form my new project will take. I was examined by the occupational doctor a few weeks ago. The part-time therapeutic return granted to me in September 2022 has just been renewed for September 2023. Let's hope this time my return goes smoothly in a lecture hall, not an operating room.

Now that my mind is better, my body is better, and my family is able to return to our small life habits. I missed it so much—the Sunday morning bike ride in the charming historic district of Old Lille! My little one has fun at the playground of the Notre-Dame de Loos abbey. Sometimes we enjoy a lemon Perrier on the terrace and buy delicious chocolate éclairs for lunch at the local pastry shop. These are all small joys I had sorely missed, and whose value I had never fully appreciated until they were abruptly taken away from me.

Every day now, I walk for almost an hour to warm up, then continue with a thirty-minute physiotherapy program. But today, it is time to no longer postpone what both excites and scares me: yoga. You now know my determination when I have a goal in mind. Over the weekend, with the help of my partner, I rearranged our room to make it a true cocoon conducive to yoga practice. Decoration, lighting, ambiance—everything is perfect! Miracles can be accomplished with a few decorative objects, a bit of paint, and four mirrors bought on *Le Bon Coin*.

For centuries, the virtues of yoga have been advocated by yoga masters and, more recently, endorsed by neuroscience. I see my return to yoga as a source of benefits on both the physical level (relaxation of muscle tension, core strength, stretching, flexibility, and muscle strengthening) and the psychological and spiritual levels (stress reduction, grounding, creativity, optimism, and serenity). These are some of the promises of yoga, and I am convinced that the philosophy of this practice can help alleviate my two types of pain. My back is now healed, so I must overcome the apprehension related to my fear of movement—the last barrier preventing complete recovery. As for my neuropathic pains in the left foot, they may always be unpredictable. I am learning to face sensations of tingling, burning, cold, numbness, hypersensitivity, and temporary paralysis with resilience.

When I put yoga back at the center of my daily life, I realize that the "Eight Limbs of Yoga" by Patañjali and the path to healing converge. At each stage, with each "limb," I grow, learn to know myself, and free myself. Yoga goes far beyond physical practice. Unfortunately, its Westernization has sometimes distorted its essence by transforming this holistic discipline—which harmoniously takes into account the totality of the individual—into a demonstration of flexibility (and often physical beauty) on social networks. However, yoga is neither a sport, gymnastics, nor a religion. It is a philosophy of life.

On the psychological level, I followed the first two limbs of yoga without initially knowing it. The *yamas* embody self-control and moral duty. To heal, changing my perception of the world was crucial. I am no longer constantly in conflict with stress, conflicts, or external elements. Thus, I could welcome what happens to me as an opportunity for self-development. Then, the *niyamas* advocate moral observance and discipline. They place me back at the heart of my life, so I offer myself the time and benevolence necessary to heal.

According to Patañjali, it is essential to live in accordance with the *yamas* and *niyamas* to prepare the mind and body for the physical practice of the third limb: *āsanas,* or postures. Paradoxically, it is the first time in my life, since I started practicing yoga, that I am truly in the right frame of mind to continue my yogic journey. The postures aim to harmonize the physical, cognitive, emotional, mental, and spiritual aspects. Thanks to them, I will continue my rehabilitation, reconnect with my bodily sensations, and regain confidence in the motor capacities of my body.

There are more than sixty shades of yoga. However, regardless of the chosen type, it is experienced in the body and especially in the mind, as it allows the restoration of the damaged mind-body connection and the reduction of short- and long-term pain (*PLOS One, September 2020*).

The fourth limb, *prāṇāyāma* or "breath," helps me detach from pain. The fifth, *pratyāhāra* or "withdrawal of the senses," teaches me to channel my senses and prevent them from scattering. The sixth, *dhāraṇā* or "concentration," brings the five senses to focus on a point other than pain. The seventh, *dhyāna* or "meditation," allows me to focus on my true self by letting the incessant flow of thoughts pass without attachment. I detach from emotions and fear. Without fear, I have no pain. The last limb is "contemplation" or *samādhi,* which I have already mentioned through Osho's narrative of his enlightenment.

But still far from seeking enlightenment, I first turn to yoga nidrā or "yogic sleep." "It is a state in which you are neither asleep nor awake. If you fall asleep, it is not yoga nidrā. If you stay awake, it is not yoga nidrā either. It is a perfect therapy. It helps you become your normal and natural self." (*Satyananda, Yoga Nidra, Yoga Publications Trust, 2002.*) It is an ancient technique that guides us into deep states of conscious relaxation by shifting our awareness from the external world to our inner world. It is complete relaxation of the body, while the mind remains awake. It is practiced in *śavāsana* (*śava,* "corpse"): lying on my back, eyes closed, the physical body silent and still, the mind at rest, and breathing gentle and effortless. I calm my mind, breath, and senses.

Let's just say things don't exactly start on a high note. It may seem easy, yet I face a major problem: I have extreme back pain. No matter how many cushions I use under my neck or knees, I can't relax into the moment. I sometimes even have to ask for help to get up. In reality, it is not so simple to let go and "unplug" the brain. I am so stressed that my fear triggers excruciating pain. It will take me several weeks of concentration and letting go to manage a complete one-hour session of yoga nidrā. In daily life, I now use this yogic sleep to alleviate my foot pain and compensate for the lack of sleep caused by my daughter's night terrors.

Indeed, according to studies, an hour of yoga nidrā brings the same benefits as four hours of sleep. A study shows that after six months of practice, 81% of practitioners experienced a reduction in headaches, gastrointestinal disorders, and back pain, allowing them to reduce their use of painkillers. Even if you are not drawn to traditional yoga, yoga nidrā can be an ally for well-being and daily sleep (*Presbyterian University College Hospital, Pittsburgh*).

Feeling initially unable to unroll my yoga mat, I opted for chair yoga, which I had also trained in. While it may be less glamorous, it proved to be an excellent compromise to start. This form of yoga works on mobility and dissipates tension. Combined with breathing and visualization techniques, a chair yoga session has been my asset for getting back in motion. I sit at the edge of my chair, both feet firmly on the ground, upright, stable, and available. I use full breathing and meditate, gently stretching my neck, cervical spine, shoulders, back, chest, hips, and legs.

During the postures, which are variations of traditional yoga *āsanas*, I smile, enjoying this moment of muscle flexibility and mental relaxation. I plan to maintain a daily chair yoga session when I return to work to reduce tensions caused by prolonged sitting positions in front of screens or stacks of papers to correct. A few minutes are truly enough to feel a calming effect. At the end of each session, I record in my journal all my sensations, pleasant or not, akin to the training logs used by athletes. This way, I track my progress and plan necessary modifications to accommodate my current level of flexibility and strength. I did this for several weeks before finally returning to my mat. Later, I turned to Iyengar yoga.

This discipline, created by B. K. S. Iyengar, is rigorous and particularly suitable for rehabilitation. The practiced poses are gentle and emphasize detail, precision, and alignment, requiring great concentration. The poses are held for long periods, and I use various props such as blocks, straps, and blankets for my comfort. I gradually strengthen my muscles, improve flexibility, and increase endurance. As my body adapts, I modify the duration and intensity of the sessions. At the same time, I use visualization techniques to prepare for a return to more dynamic yoga.

What do Serena Williams, Michael Jordan, and Tiger Woods have in common? They win "in their minds" before doing it "in reality" on the courts or courses worldwide. These renowned athletes are programmed to be the best regardless of circumstances. They have experienced the cross-court forehand, the buzzer-beating jump shot, or the decisive swing. But mental imagery is not only used in sports. Arnold Schwarzenegger, former Mr. Universe, explains that he used the same methods to succeed as a bodybuilder, actor, and politician: "What you have to do is create an image of who you want to be and then visualize it as if it were already a reality." (*Schwarzenegger, Total Recall, Simon & Schuster UK, 2013.*)

Another example is James Nesmith, an average golfer who wanted to improve his game but was prevented from doing so by the Vietnam War. As a prisoner of war, he spent seven long years in a tiny cell measuring 1.5 meters by 1.8 meters. He saw no one, talked to no one, and had no physical activity. In the early months, he awaited his release. But soon, he realized that if he didn't find a way to occupy his mind, he would go mad. James Nesmith decided to play golf every day —in his head!

He visualized the scene in as much detail as possible: the feel of his clothes on his skin, the smell of freshly cut grass, the touch of the sun, and the gentle breeze on his face. Nothing was missing! Trees stood in front of him, birds sang, and squirrels jumped from branch to branch. Everything was there! He gripped his club, felt the roughness of the grip under his fingers, hit the ball, and walked to the putter. He took his club, made a few swings, and hit again. He imagined his position and felt the weight of the club in his hands. He visualized the arc of the ball in the air... And since everything was virtual, he played well and missed few shots. In a cell in Vietnam or at home? No difference for our golfer's brain.

He followed the course, playing each hole until the last, doing this for seven years, four hours a day. Upon his return to the United States, the story took a surprising turn. Even though he was physically much diminished, he returned to the green and scored 74 shots—nearly 20 shots better than his average before the war. Without touching a club for seven years, he became a good golfer.

Are you still skeptical about the power of visualization? Natan Sharansky, accused of espionage, endured a nine-year sentence in a Soviet prison. In isolation, he played chess mentally to survive. In 1996, during an exhibition, he met world chess champion Garry Kasparov, who played simultaneously against five opponents. Not surprisingly, Kasparov won four games, but to the astonishment of the crowd, lost to Sharansky: "You know, I beat him twelve times... in my head. So, I was programmed. Beating him was the most natural thing in the world for me."

Reality is only a perception. Whether I imagine an event or actually live it, the same chemical and functional reactions are triggered in my brain. Life battles are won or lost in our brains before we truly engage in them.

"There are only beautiful roads, and no matter where they lead us..."

Jean-Jacques Goldman, *On ira*, 1997.

A French example or an American one:

"Ain't about how fast I get there

Ain't about what's waiting on the other side

It's the climb..."

Miley Cyrus, *The Climb*.

Thus, over the weeks, I have embraced a new meaning of the word *success*. Success now means reconnecting with my body, breathing mindfully, feeling the fluidity of movements, savoring positive emotions and sensations, and enjoying the present moment. I have abandoned the idea of achieving lauded poses and instead prioritize poses that suit my body as it is, here and now. I appreciate the journey, not the destination. After each session, I record my sensations in a journal, allowing me to track my progress and prepare for the next session.

By adopting this approach, I connect with the original philosophy of yoga and no longer let setbacks undermine me. The *āsanas* of my session were different yesterday and will be different tomorrow. Yoga is not a performance to complete; it is an experience to live, a moment of pleasure to surrender to! Pose after pose, I rediscover my enthusiasm and free myself from fear and the tyranny of perfectionism. Thus, even if my pains continue to linger in the corner of my mind, I am happy. As the sessions progress, the residual pains fade, just like the fear I once had of them.

Cam is introduced to yoga in my company. We tease each other during balance-focused sessions—what may seem simple to achieve is not always so! Having resumed my training to become a yoga teacher, I also need to test the sessions I create. My husband helps a lot, providing his technical perspective on body alignment and the muscles involved in postures. Emily is not left behind. She requests *Moana*-themed yoga sessions, which I create for her with pleasure.

I am also the proudest of moms when she joins a virtual class I participate in. Downward Dog, Cobra, and Triangle are her favorites! She even manages to charm all the participants by performing a perfect namaste when the teacher concludes the session... What indescribable joy it is to reconnect with precious moments of serenity and happiness with her.

However, one final obstacle still awaits me: the clutch pedal of my car! Despite the neuropathic pains in my foot, thanks to rehabilitation and yoga, I have regained enough sensitivity and mobility to overcome this challenge. I will start with small errands around the corner before considering a visit to my parents twenty minutes away. Finally, in a few weeks, I will drive to the Oignies rehabilitation center thirty kilometers from home. I am independent again; the end of this long ordeal is near.

Upon reflection, success is simple to achieve. It depends on how we define it and where we place the "success" cursor. From my experience, I believe the same applies to happiness. Being happy is as simple as waking up and smiling at life. I will now be satisfied with my actions and initiatives, regardless of the final result. The time for doubts is over. I have confidence; I will be reborn and live again, peaceful, happy, and carefree. Dear brain, from now on, I am fine. Thank you!

EPILOGUE

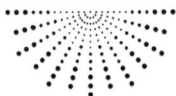

Dear Reader,

      June 12, 2023, will forever be etched in my memory as a profoundly symbolic day. Standing at the Les Hautois rehabilitation center, I was ready to resume running through a personalized program designed just for me. After two years of silence, I chose this day to share a message of hope on social media. A phrase lingers in my mind, spoken timidly, with palpable emotion and tears welling in the corners of her eyes by my daughter:

"Is it true? Can you carry me now, Mummy?"

After four weeks of rehabilitation, this phrase embodies my triumph over chronic pain. Believe me, one day you will see, that by carrying this being in your arms, the answers to all your questions will find you.

But believe me, one day you will see,
As you hold this being, pure and free,
All your doubts will fade, so let it be...

Our body is a virtuoso of adaptation! When rebellion brews, we must find ways to release the overflow of stress and emotions before the storm breaks and our glass overflows.

Day after day, you have accompanied me on this journey to rediscover tools that prevent fear from dictating my life. With my toolbox now full, I can embrace life with confidence, filling my glass without fear of it spilling over. I am finally living my best life, aligned with my passions and values, listening to the signals of my body, which will always guide me to stay in my pain-free zone. I will cultivate enthusiasm, gratitude, and daily joy, nurturing my mental image and cherishing my brain.

Writing this testimony was not easy. Revisiting these painful memories often brought nightmares and emotional turmoil. Reliving each trial was a profound challenge, but it also allowed me to close the chapter of suffering and begin a new one filled with hope and possibility. I never believed such a transformation was possible when I struggled to regain full use of my left side.

I hope my story has surprised you, revealing the incredible power of the body–mind connection. I hope it has challenged your certainties and opened your eyes to the untapped strength and resilience within each of us. Chronic pain exposed my ignorance—despite devouring countless personal development books over the years, I now realize I understood little. Our true enemy is fear. Insidious and lurking, it prevents us from fully experiencing our emotions and potential.

Even if you do not suffer from chronic pain, you have your own battles. My wish is that this story makes you aware of the immense strength and resilience lying dormant within you.

The persistent neuropathic pain in my left foot, a remnant of my past paralysis, continues to oscillate between intense and moderate. Day by day, I am learning to tame it. I now accept it as part of me—a witness to my ordeal and a reminder of everything I have endured: the good, the bad, and the transformative.

At the rehabilitation center, thanks to the creativity of my occupational therapist, I reconnected with my passion for surfing. All that remains now is to use visualization to mentally prepare for real conditions and to overcome the lifelong fear of water that has haunted me. Soon, the waves will be mine.

With gratitude and hope,

Lili Road

NOTES

CHAPTER 25

1. (Kim et al., *"Emotional, motivational and interpersonal responsiveness of children with autism in improvisational music therapy,"* Autism., 2009.)

ACKNOWLEDGMENTS

Camille, from the bottom of my heart, a huge thank you for your patience and invaluable contribution to this testimony. I am deeply grateful to have had you by my side to face the highs and lows of this human and artistic adventure. Without you, nothing would have been possible. I remember each of our passionate discussions about every comma and nuance of meaning. This shared passion defines us, and I eagerly look forward to seeing where our next journey will lead us.

Emily, Mathilde, Alex, I send you all my love. You are a source of daily happiness, and I am immensely proud to be your mother. I also think of Noah and Thomas. Mom, Dad, thank you for instilling in me a thirst for learning and the values of altruism that I strive to practice every day. Thank you for supporting me through every career change and each time I decided to resume my studies. Your unwavering belief in me has allowed me to reach where I am today.

Thank you, Barry and Sandra—I love you forever. To my Canadian parents, brothers, and sisters: thank you for giving me the time of my life. You'll always be in my heart. I warmly thank the members of the Rotary Club and Lions Club in France and Canada.

Mrs. Hanssens and Dr. Nectoux, I want to express my gratitude to you both—you sparked a vocation in me. Professor Sarno, thank you for opening my eyes to a pain-free world. Doctors Schubiner and Gordon, I thank you both for your time and trust in my research.

Dr. Delattre, Dr. Wieczorek, Dr. Zairi, Mr. Grosdemouge, Mr. Gosselin, Charlotte, Mrs. Psychologist, and the entire team at the medico-psychological center—I sincerely thank you for your unwavering support.

To my friends Christine, Julie, Diane, and Hélène; Elsie, Wendy, and Lucinda: warm hugs to you all. Through bad times and good times, you were there no matter what! Michelle, my dearest friend, I miss you and can't wait to see you again! A heartfelt thought for Flavie, Paul, and Hugo.

Thank you to you, the audience, who inspired me to write songs and create. And to you, dear readers, for reading this book and perhaps even lending it to others.

I also want to thank Frédéric Veille for his support and advice, as well as City Éditions for their trust.

Finally, I'd like to express my deepest gratitude to Usher and Library Tales Publishing. After speaking with you, I realized how fortunate I was that our paths crossed. Thank you for placing your trust in me!

From the depths of my heart, thank you!

Now, I find myself facing a dilemma: it is impossible for me to mention everyone who deserves recognition in these acknowledgments. To those who recognize themselves, I dedicate this testimony with all the gratitude it contains.

As I write this page today, September 11, exactly one year after my surgery, I am fully immersed in what I cherish and what I call the "gratitude attitude."

www.ingramcontent.com/pod-product-compliance
Lightning Source LLC
LaVergne TN
LVHW012341050925
819951LV00007B/27